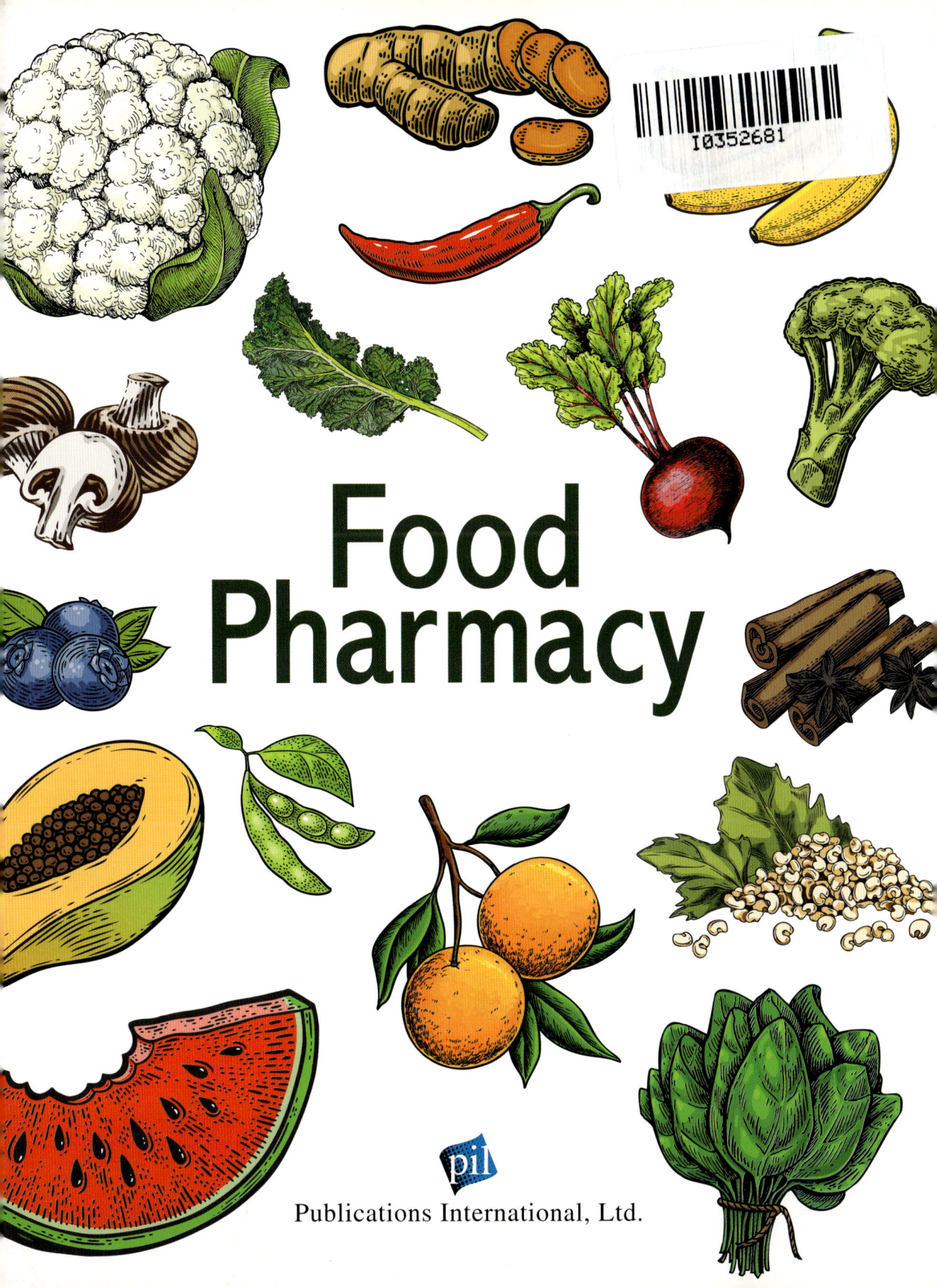

Food Pharmacy

Publications International, Ltd.

Images from Shutterstock.com

Copyright © 2024 Publications International, Ltd. All rights reserved. This book may not be reproduced or quoted in whole or in part by any means whatsoever without written permission from:

Louis Weber, CEO
Publications International, Ltd.
8140 Lehigh Avenue
Morton Grove, IL 60053

Permission is never granted for commercial purposes.

ISBN: 978-1-63938-543-0

Manufactured in China.

8 7 6 5 4 3 2 1

This publication is only intended to provide general information. The information is specifically not intended to substitute for medical diagnosis or treatment by your physician or other healthcare professional. You should always consult your own physician or other healthcare professionals about any medical questions, diagnosis, or treatment. (Products vary among manufacturers. Please check labels carefully to confirm that the products you use are appropriate for your condition.)

The information obtained by you from this publication should not be relied upon for any personal, nutritional, or medical decision. You should consult an appropriate professional for specific advice tailored to your specific situation. PIL makes no representation or warranties, express or implied, with respect to your use of this information.

In no event shall PIL or its affiliates or advertisers be liable for any direct, indirect, punitive, incidental, special, or consequential damages, or any damages whatsoever including, without limitation, damages for personal injury, death, damage to property or loss of profits, arising out of or in any way connected with the use of any of the above-referenced information or otherwise arising out of use of this publication.

Let's get social!
@Publications_International
@PublicationsInternational
www.pilbooks.com

CONTENTS

Introduction 4
Vitamins and Minerals for Prevention 6
Anti-Inflammatory Foods 38
Putting It All Together 52
Conditions 74

Allergies 74
Alzheimer's Disease 76
Anemia 80
Anxiety 83
Arthritis 86
Asthma 88
Back Pain 90
Belching 91
Bronchitis 93
Canker Sores 95
Colds 97
Cold Sores 99
Colic 101
Constipation 103
Cough 105
Dehydration 107
Diabetes 109
Diarrhea 113
Dry Mouth 115
Fever 117
Flatulence 119
Flu (Influenza) 122
Food Poisoning 124
Foot Discomfort and Odor 125

Gallbladder Problems 127
Gout 130
Hangovers 134
Heartburn 137
Heart Disease 141
High Blood Pressure 143
High Cholesterol 145
Insomnia 148
Irritable Bowel Syndrome 151
Lactose Intolerance 154
Low Immunity 158
Menopause 161
Menstrual Problems 163
Motion Sickness 165
Muscle Soreness and Cramping . 167
Osteoporosis 170
Poor Appetite 173
Premenstrual Syndrome 176
Seasonal Affective Disorder 179
Sore Throat 182
Stomach Upset 185
Ulcers 189
Urinary Tract Infection 191

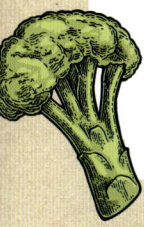
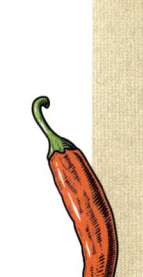

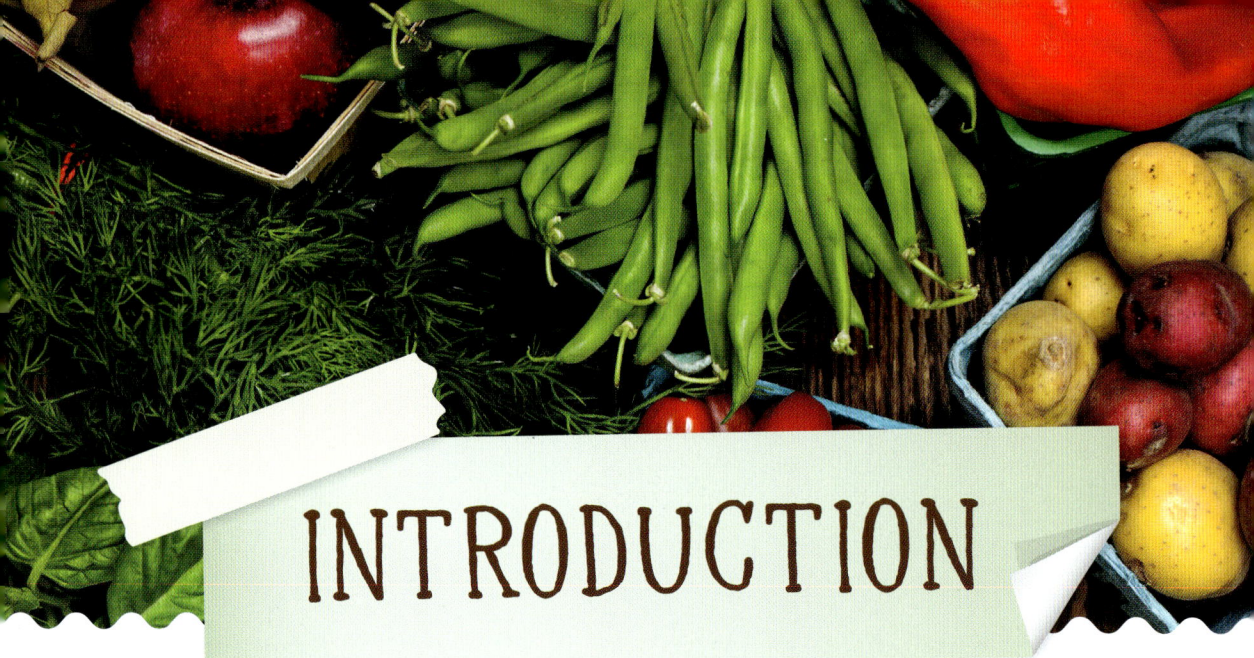

INTRODUCTION

Many of the most common health problems we face today—from annoying problems like constipation to more serious conditions such as heart disease—are linked to what we eat. Within the last several decades, the focus of research into possible links between nutrition and health has expanded; it now includes not only the potential dangers of eating certain foods (or too much of certain foods) but also the natural healing and protective powers that some foods possess.

That's not to say that food alone can cure disease or take the place of medical treatment. It is, however, becoming increasingly evident that food has disease-fighting potential. Translation? You have the power to choose foods that may help prevent and treat a host of today's most common maladies.

The more we research, the more proof we have: Eating well and good health are intertwined. Eating right can't prevent or cure every illness—but eating nutrient-dense foods that give us the vitamins and minerals we need is necessary for good long-term health. More than that, for a number of chronic conditions, including certain foods in your diet—or excluding others—can help soothe symptoms, forestall further health problems, and even reverse the progression of the disease.

In **Food Pharmacy**, you will find information about how food interacts with more than forty health conditions. Some, like colds and stomach upset, are short-term problems. What you eat during that time can help you ride out the unpleasantness and provide fast relief for symptoms. In other cases, for chronic conditions like diabetes and heart disease, your long-term food choices are critical to your management of the disease. You'll also find information about the vitamins you need, the best dietary choices for long-term heart health and cognitive functioning, and the ins and outs of anti-inflammatory foods.

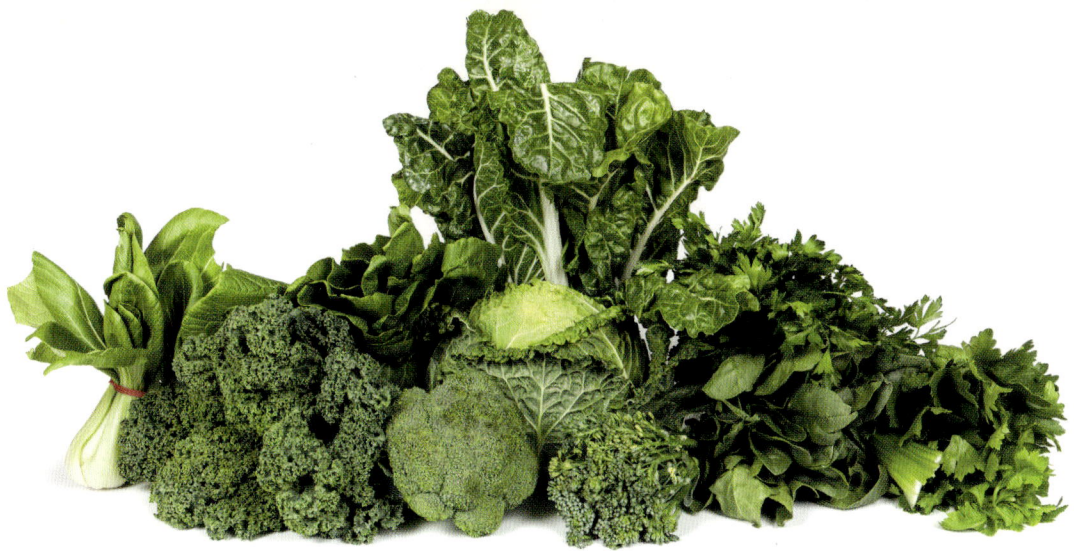

THE BEST DIET?

We often wonder what to eat to maintain optimum health. To some extent the answers are personal. Bodies are different, and the best diet for you will be the one that gives you the most energy and makes you feel the best. However, we do know some general guidelines for eating for good health:

- Eat meals heavy on vegetables, fruits, and grains.

- Eat an array of vegetables, in all colors. For leafy green vegetables, the darker the green, the more nutrients are available.

- Eat red meat sparingly.

- Eat fish a few times each week. Fatty fish like salmon and tuna carry an array of health benefits.

- Every so often, we hear about a new "superfood." Many are overhyped—no single food is a miracle food—but yogurt, berries, salmon, dark leafy greens, and beans and other legumes are all packed with nutrients and offer a variety of health benefits.

GETTING STARTED

When it comes to putting healing medicine in an easy-to-swallow package, Mother Nature has truly outdone science. Fortunately, science is catching on and gradually uncovering the many ways that food, especially food in its natural state, appears able to help the body heal and protect itself. With the aid of **Food Pharmacy**, you can put that newly discovered knowledge to work for your own health's sake, with each food you choose and each bite you take.

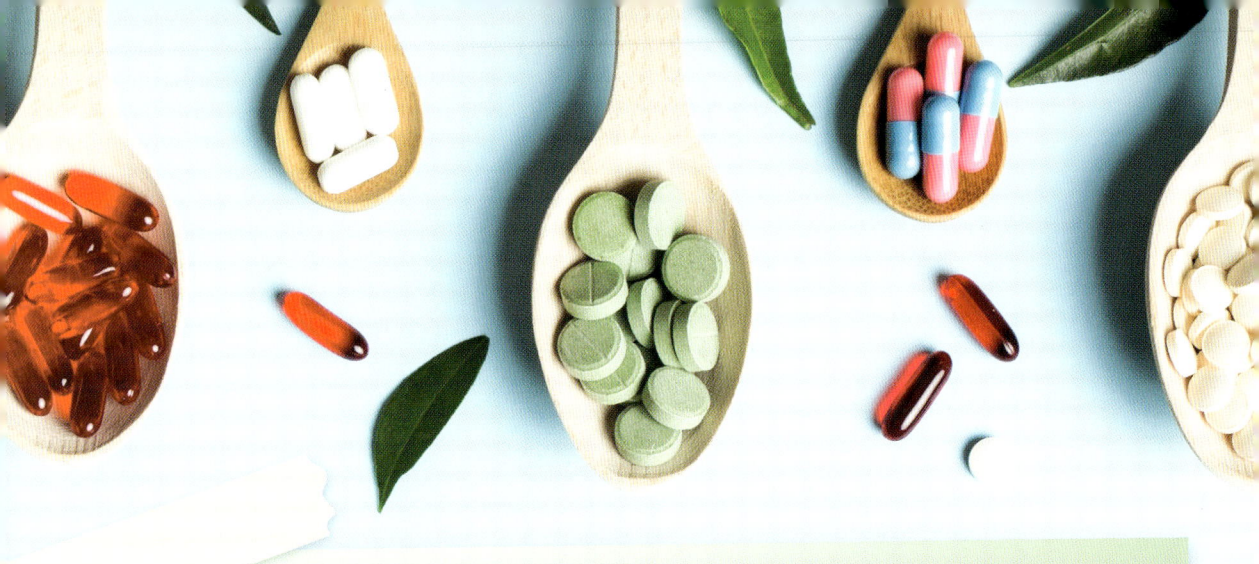

VITAMINS AND MINERALS FOR PREVENTION

Getting enough of essential nutrients is a good start on the road to a healthy immune system that staves off illnesses and chronic diseases. Generally, eating a well-balanced diet will get you on that road. A healthy diet provides you with an assortment of necessary vitamins and minerals, in the quantities you need to maintain health.

What Are Vitamins?

Vitamins are organic substances that are necessary in very small amounts to maintain normal metabolism in the body. The phrase "in very small amounts" included in the definition sets vitamins apart from the other classes of essential organic compounds. For example, proteins, fats, and carbohydrates are also organic substances, but we require them in considerably greater quantities. We measure vitamins in milligrams (mg) and micrograms (mcg or µg); in contrast, we measure proteins, fats, and carbohydrates in grams (g).

We've only known about the existence of vitamins since 1912. Since that time, scientists have identified approximately 13 vitamins. The last to be isolated was vitamin B12 in the late 1940s. Upon its discovery, researchers assigned a letter designation to each vitamin in alphabetical order. It turned out, however, that some of the vitamins were actually several substances. The compound vitamin B, for example, turned out to be a group of compounds. So we now have vitamin B1, vitamin B2, vitamin B6, and so forth. Although vitamins' alphabetical designations are still in common use, they also have chemical names.

All vitamins are essential to life and must be supplied in the diet. As with any rule, though, there are exceptions. The body does produce small amounts of biotin, vitamin B12, and vitamin K from intestinal bacteria, but in such negligible quantities that we still need more from the foods we eat.

Vitamin	Chemical Name(s)
Vitamin A	Beta-carotene; retinol
Vitamin B1	Thiamine
Vitamin B2	Riboflavin
Vitamin B3	Niacin; niacinamide
Vitamin B5	Pantothenic acid
Vitamin B6	Pyridoxine; pyridoxamine; pyridoxal
Vitamin B7	Biotin
Vitamin B9	Folic acid; folate
Vitamin B12	Cobalamin; cyanocobalamin; hydroxycobalamin; methylcobalamin
Vitamin C	Ascorbic acid
Vitamin D	Cholecalciferol (D3); ergocalciferol (D2)
Vitamin E	Tocopherol; tocotrienols
Vitamin K	Menadione (K3); menaquinone (K2); phylloquinone, phytomenadione, phytonadione (K1)

Furthermore, if the body is supplied with the proper raw materials, it is capable of manufacturing certain other vitamins. For example, plant foods such as fruits and vegetables don't actually contain vitamin A but instead have vitamin A "activity." In other words, they are "precursors" to vitamin A because they contain substances called carotenes that our bodies can convert to vitamin A. Carotenoid is the substance that makes certain fruits and vegetables yellow, orange, or red. Some carotenoids, such as beta-carotene, alpha-carotene, and beta-cryptoxanthin, can be made into vitamin A by the body. Other carotenoids, such as lycopene, lutein, and zeaxanthin, cannot be made into vitamin A by the body. All carotenoids are antioxidants. These precursors are sometimes called provitamin A. Carotenes may also function as antioxidants, giving them importance beyond their conversion to vitamin A.

We have a provitamin D in our skin. Sunlight triggers a chemical reaction in skin that begins the provitamin's complex conversion to vitamin D—a process that is later completed in the kidneys. This explains vitamin D's nickname, the "sunshine vitamin." Often, though, the amount produced this way isn't enough to meet our bodies' needs, and we still need a dietary source. The body also meets some of its niacin needs by conversion from the amino acid tryptophan. Because we must rely on diet to fulfill our requirements for these vitamins, they are all essential.

WATER-SOLUBLE VS. FAT-SOLUBLE

One way to classify vitamins is by solubility. Water-soluble vitamins—the B vitamins and vitamin C—dissolve in water. Water-soluble vitamins can't be stored in the body, so you need them more frequently. Excess vitamins are excreted in urine. Water-soluble vitamins are mainly found in fruits and vegetables, grains, and milk and dairy foods.

Fat-soluble vitamins—A, D, E, and K—require fat for absorption. Fat-soluble vitamins are mainly found in animal fats, vegetable oils, dairy foods, liver, and oily fish. While your body needs these vitamins to work properly, you don't need to eat foods containing them every day.

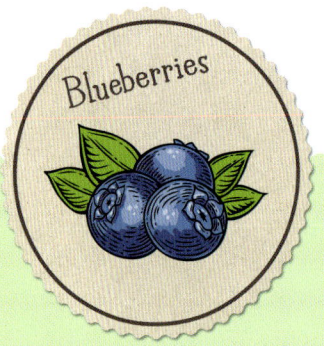

WHAT ARE ANTIOXIDANTS?

Our bodies need oxygen, but if an oxygen molecule loses one of its electrons, it becomes an unstable, destructive free radical that assaults healthy cells in order to try to get its missing electron back. Classes of molecular compounds called antioxidants neutralize free radicals and shield healthy cells. Some vitamins and minerals are antioxidants. Special chemicals in plants called phytochemicals can also act as antioxidants. We can arm ourselves with these natural protective chemicals by eating a diet rich in plant foods.

LOTS FROM LITTLE

Many vitamins, especially those of the B complex, act as coenzymes, or small molecules attached to enzymes that help the enzymes do their job. An enzyme is a catalyst—a substance that regulates the speed of a chemical reaction without being used up or changed in that reaction. So our bodies can use enzymes over and over again to control specific reactions. The body can also repeatedly use vitamins that act as coenzymes. However, the body still needs a regular supply of these and the other vitamins to replace those excreted in the urine or destroyed or changed by the body during certain metabolic processes.

DEFICIENCIES

Vitamin deficiencies have been linked to all sorts of health problems, including heart disease, anemia, osteoporosis, scurvy, rickets, and cancer. Fortunately, serious vitamin deficiencies are rare in the United States today. Concern about vitamin deficiencies is rapidly being replaced with concern about the effects of marginally adequate vitamin intakes—amounts that may not cause a vitamin-deficiency disease but might interfere with normal body functions.

A subclinical deficiency can sneak up on you when the amount of a nutrient in your diet or your total "body pool" of a nutrient is only marginally adequate. Biochemical and metabolic changes can begin to take place, and then you become at risk for a vitamin deficiency. Waiting to act on your nutrient needs until you have a clear deficiency or a disease is not a prudent approach.

One way to protect yourself from the dangers of undetectable subclinical deficiencies is to eat a wide variety of foods. If you do not eat enough calories, or if your eating habits are not as good as you would like, you may want to consider taking a multivitamin mineral supplement. The supplement should balance what you are already getting from your diet. Always consult your doctor before starting any supplements.

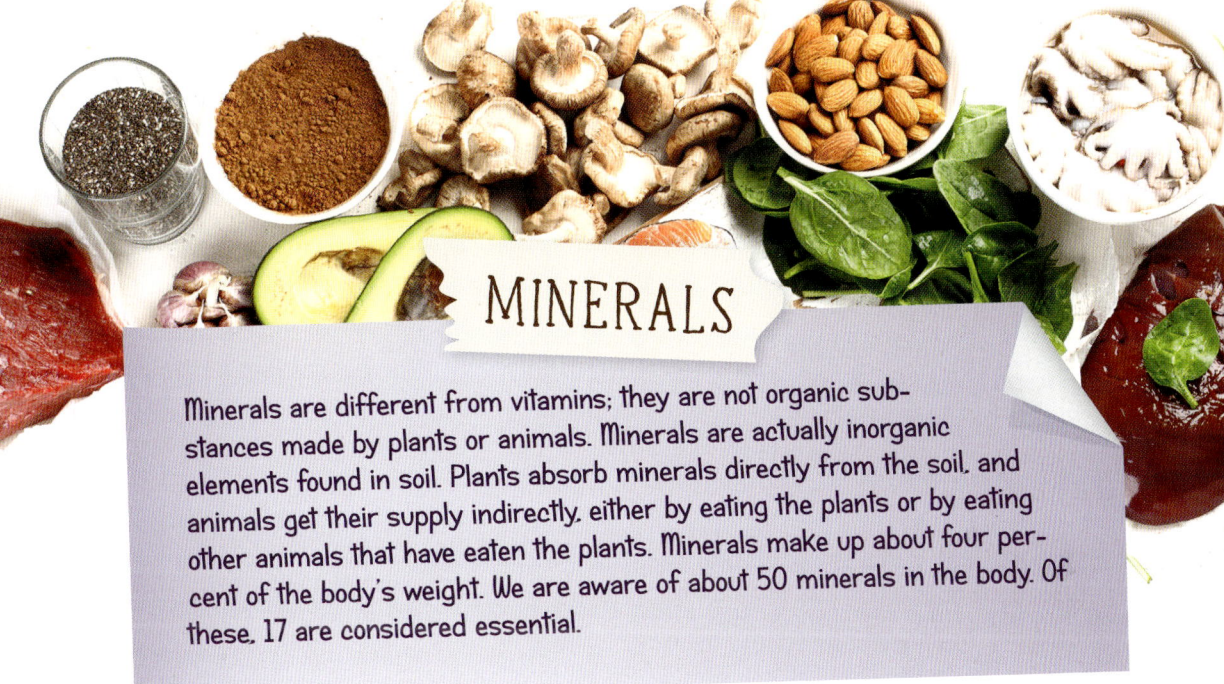

MINERALS

Minerals are different from vitamins; they are not organic substances made by plants or animals. Minerals are actually inorganic elements found in soil. Plants absorb minerals directly from the soil, and animals get their supply indirectly, either by eating the plants or by eating other animals that have eaten the plants. Minerals make up about four percent of the body's weight. We are aware of about 50 minerals in the body. Of these, 17 are considered essential.

There are two kinds of minerals—macrominerals and trace minerals. Minerals are grouped into these two categories depending on the amount found in the body. You need larger amounts of macrominerals (also called major minerals). They include calcium, phosphorus, magnesium, sodium, potassium, chloride, and sulfur. You only need small amounts of trace minerals (also called microminerals). They include iron, manganese, copper, iodine, zinc, cobalt, fluoride, and selenium.

For many trace minerals, there is a fine line between not enough and too much. Most of the benefits attributed to minerals come from consuming the normal amounts found in foods. Unless you are correcting a deficiency under a doctor's supervision, taking more than the recommended amount of a mineral may do more harm than good.

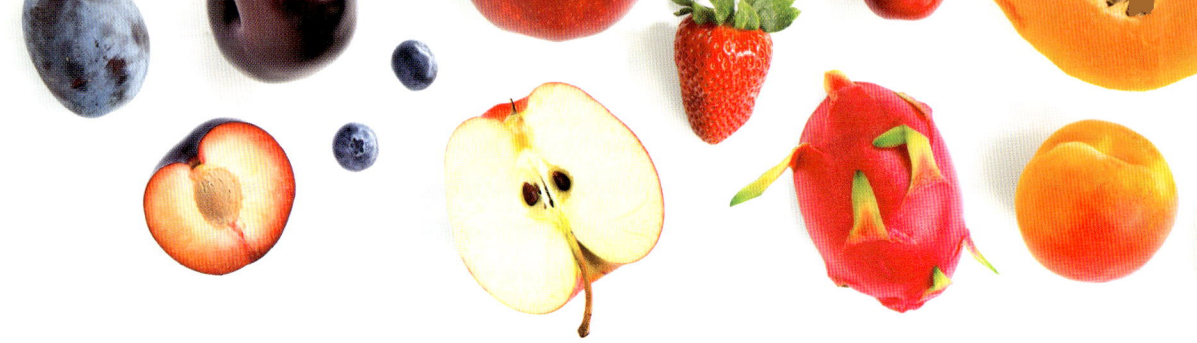

Macrominerals	Trace Minerals
Calcium	Chromium
Chloride	Cobalt
Magnesium	Copper
Phosphorus	Fluoride
Potassium	Iodine
Sodium	Iron
Sulfur	Manganese
	Molybdenum
	Selenium
	Zinc

WHAT MINERALS DO

Did you know that every cell in the body contains minerals? In fact, almost everything the body does involves minerals in some way or another. Their main functions are to help maintain the structure of living tissue and to regulate important body processes.

In their structural role, minerals contribute strength and firmness to bones and teeth. They're also part of essential body compounds. For example, iron is a part of hemoglobin (the oxygen-carrying substance in red blood cells) and is also a part of a number of different enzymes; iodine is a part of the thyroid hormone; and cobalt is a part of vitamin B12.

In their role as regulators, minerals act as cofactors in enzyme-controlled body reactions. In other words, they keep enzyme reactions running up to speed. Iron, zinc, and copper are parts of enzymes. If the diet doesn't supply enough of these minerals, the body can't make enough enzymes.

DEFICIENCIES

Nutrition surveys occasionally find that intake of certain minerals, such as calcium, potassium, iron, and zinc, are lower than recommended. A mineral deficiency often happens slowly over time.

Common causes of deficiencies include an increased need for the mineral, lack of the mineral in the diet, or difficulty absorbing the mineral from food. Many food manufacturers replace some of the minerals lost during processing—a process called enrichment. In the 1920s, health authorities successfully prevented iodine-deficiency goiter by adding iodine to salt. Manufacturers frequently add iron to cereals and breads that have the mineral stripped during processing. Many companies add calcium to fruit juices, breakfast cereals, and breads, too. The best way to prevent or remedy nutrient deficiencies is to eat a balanced, nutrient-rich diet.

Food vs. Supplements

Wouldn't it be nice to meet all your nutritional needs by swallowing a single pill? Unfortunately, it doesn't work that way. Supplements, by definition, are there to supplement a diet, not substitute for it. Food is essential to good health. Although we know something about food and the components that are vital to good health, we will never know everything. For example, scientists have already identified more than 10,000 non-nutrient compounds in plant foods. Each has shown some positive effects on health.

Food is also preferable to supplements as a primary source of vitamins and minerals because it's much more difficult to get too much of a substance from food, making overdosing unlikely. Talk with your health care provider before taking any high doses typical of megadose supplements, as the drug-like effects of nutrients can be harmful. Although toxicity rarely causes death, it can cause considerable discomfort and interfere with the healthy functioning of the body.

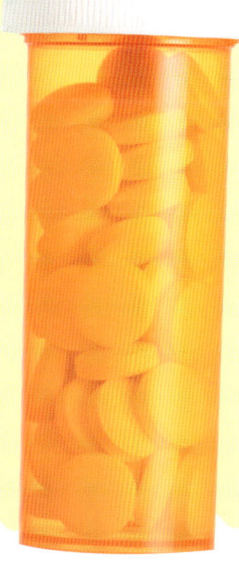

TAKING CARE

Nutritional supplements range from the familiar vitamins and minerals to herbal remedies. Each can support good health and help prevent and treat various disorders. Remember, though, that just because a substance is natural does not mean it can't be harmful. In excess or under certain conditions, many natural substances can be toxic. That's why it's important not to self-diagnose. If you are using prescription medications, tell all your doctors about every supplement and medication you take. Decide on a dosage that is safe for you in consultation with your health care providers.

Now that we've looked at the general role that vitamins and minerals play, let's look at specifics.

VITAMIN A
(Beta-Carotene)

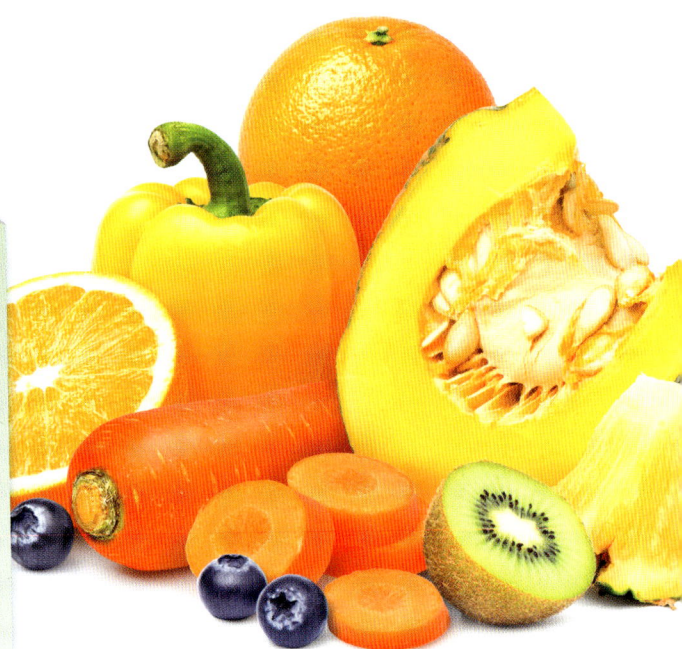

Beta-carotene is one of a group of red, orange, and yellow pigments called carotenoids. The body converts beta-carotene into vitamin A, an essential nutrient needed for healthy eyes and skin, normal growth and development, and immune system function. Like all carotenoids, beta-carotene is an antioxidant. Antioxidants help fight against free radicals.

SOURCES OF BETA-CAROTENE

Beta-carotene is found in orange, red, and yellow plant foods and in some dark green vegetables. Good sources of beta-carotene include carrots, sweet potatoes, pumpkin, collard greens, spinach, kale, broccoli, winter squash, cantaloupe, and apricots.

Carrots

SUPPLEMENTS

Beta-carotene is included in some antioxidant and multivitamin supplements, and is also available in separate beta-carotene supplements. Beta-carotene supplements are not recommended for general use. Don't take beta-carotene supplements if you smoke.

BETA-CAROTENE AND HEALTH

Beta-carotene can reduce sun sensitivity in people with erythropoietic protoporphyria, an inherited blood disorder. Beta-carotene may also help prevent age-related macular degeneration, breast cancer, pregnancy-related complications, and sunburn.

While people who eat a lot of foods containing beta-carotene might have a lower risk of certain kinds of cancer, studies have not yet shown that vitamin A or beta-carotene supplements can help prevent cancer.

B VITAMINS

B vitamins are a group of water-soluble vitamins that are important for cell function. The B vitamins are: thiamin (vitamin B1), riboflavin (vitamin B2), niacin (vitamin B3), pantothenic acid (vitamin B5), vitamin B6, biotin (vitamin B7), folate (vitamin B9), and vitamin B12. These eight vitamins make up the vitamin B complex. B vitamins are found in yeast, seeds, eggs, liver, meat, and vegetables.

Eggs

VITAMIN B1 (Thiamin)

Like other B-complex vitamins, thiamin acts as a biological catalyst, or coenzyme. As a coenzyme, thiamin participates in the long chain of reactions that provides energy for the body and heat. Thiamin helps the body manufacture fats and metabolize protein. It's also needed for normal functioning of the nervous system.

SOURCES OF THIAMIN

Thiamin is naturally found in some foods and added to other food products. Enriched breads and cereals, meat (especially pork), fish, legumes, seeds, nuts, and whole grains are good sources of thiamin. Most other foods, fruits, and dairy products contain only small amounts of thiamin.

Heating foods containing thiamin at high temperatures can reduce their thiamin content. As a water-soluble vitamin, thiamin also tends to leach out of food into the cooking water. In order to preserve thiamin, it's best to cook food over low temperatures in small amounts of water for short periods. Steaming and microwaving can help minimize losses of thiamin and preserve the natural flavors of the foods.

Sulfites, used as preservatives, also destroy thiamin. Your best bet for preserving a food's thiamin content is to use additives sparingly and keep the cooking time short.

THIAMIN DEFICIENCY

A thiamin deficiency can develop if the body eliminates too much or absorbs too little thiamin, or if there's insufficient thiamin in the diet. Diets deficient in thiamin are often deficient in other B vitamins as well.

Vitamins and Minerals for Prevention

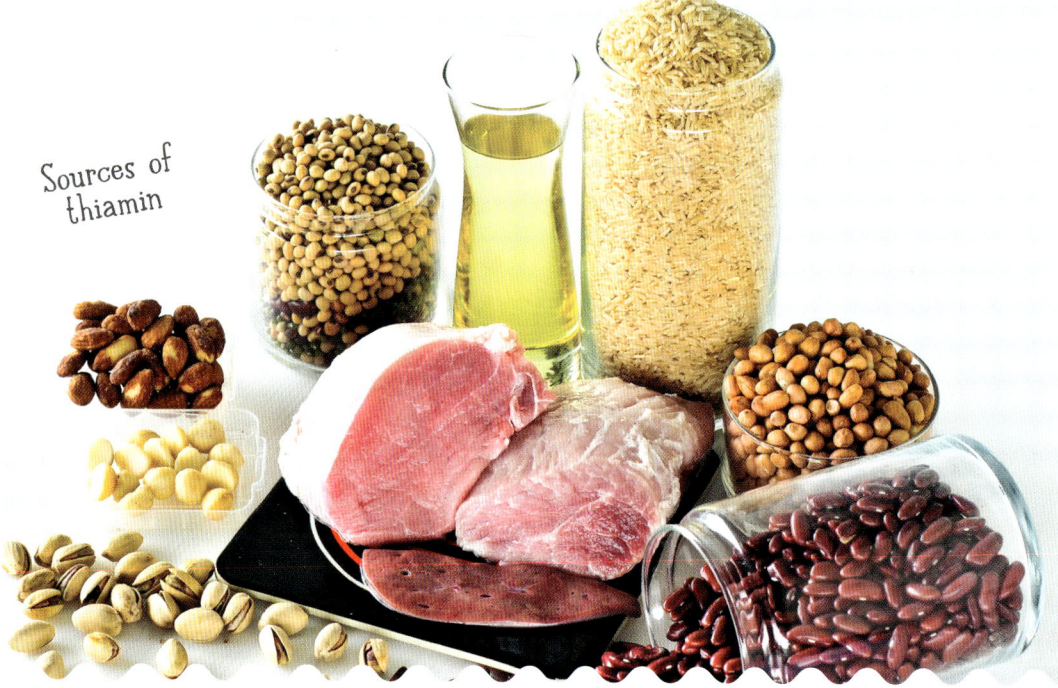

Sources of thiamin

Signs and symptoms of thiamin deficiency include weight loss, loss of appetite, confusion, memory loss, muscle weakness, and heart problems. Severe thiamin deficiency leads to a serious disease called beriberi disease with the added symptoms of tingling and numbness in the feet and hands, muscle loss, and poor reflexes.

THIAMIN AND HEALTH

Thiamin supplements are used for a variety of potential health benefits. In addition to helping prevent and treat thiamin deficiency, thiamin has been shown to help correct certain inherited metabolic disorders. Thiamin also seems to help decrease the risk and symptoms of the brain disorder Wernicke-Korsakoff syndrome, which is often seen in alcoholics. It causes tingling and numbness in the hands and feet, severe memory loss, disorientation, and confusion.

VITAMIN B2
(Riboflavin)

Riboflavin is important for cell growth, development, and function. It also helps turn food into energy. Riboflavin acts as a coenzyme—the non-protein, active portion of an enzyme—by helping to metabolize carbohydrates, fats, and proteins to provide the body with energy. Riboflavin doesn't act alone, however; it works in concert with its B-complex relatives. Riboflavin also plays a role in the metabolism of other vitamins.

SOURCES OF RIBOFLAVIN

Riboflavin is found naturally in some foods and is added to many fortified foods. Eggs, organ meats, lean meats, and milk are particularly rich in riboflavin. Green vegetables such as asparagus, broccoli, and spinach also provide some riboflavin. Riboflavin is added to many fortified cereals, breads, and grain products. The daily value (DV) for riboflavin, which was established by the FDA, is 1.7 milligrams for adults and children age 4 and older.

PROTECT YOUR RIBOFLAVIN

Milk in plastic jugs is more susceptible to loss of riboflavin and vitamin A than milk in paperboard cartons. That's because light, even the fluorescent light in supermarkets, destroys these two light-sensitive nutrients.

RIBOFLAVIN DEFICIENCY

Most people in the United States get enough riboflavin from the foods they eat and deficiencies are extremely rare. Riboflavin deficiency can cause skin disorders, sores at the corners of the mouth, swollen and cracked lips, hair loss, sore throat, liver disorders, and problems with the reproductive and nervous systems. Anemia and cataracts can develop if riboflavin deficiency is severe and prolonged.

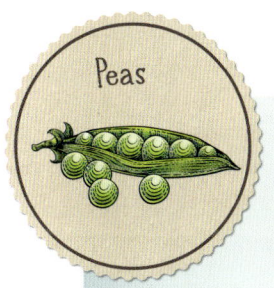

VITAMIN B3
(Niacin)

The body needs niacin to convert food into energy, and to keep the nervous system, digestive tract, and skin healthy. Niacin is used to lower high blood pressure and cholesterol, and to treat niacin deficiency.

SOURCES OF NIACIN

Niacin is found in foods such as yeast, milk and other dairy products, eggs, lean meats, poultry, fish, legumes, nuts, and whole grains. Many breads and breakfast cereals are also fortified with niacin during the manufacturing process.

NIACIN DEFICIENCY

Pellagra is a disease of deficiency of niacin (vitamin B3). It can result from an inability to absorb niacin or the amino acid tryptophan. The first symptoms of pellagra are weakness, loss of appetite, and some digestive disturbances. As the deficiency disease progresses, the skin becomes rough and red in areas exposed to sunlight, heat, or irritation. Later, open sores, diarrhea, dementia, and delirium may develop. Death results if the condition is left untreated.

This disease, now rarely seen in the United States, is still common in parts of the world where corn is the major cereal grain. Corn is deficient in tryptophan, and the niacin it contains is difficult to absorb. In many Latin American countries, they combine cornmeal with the mineral lime when making tortillas; the alkalinity of the lime frees the niacin so that it can be absorbed.

NIACIN USE AND MISUSE

Treatment for niacin deficiency commonly involves giving 25 to 50 milligrams (mg) of the vitamin daily. Larger doses of one form of niacin, nicotinic acid, in amounts ranging from 500 milligrams (mg) to 3 grams (g) daily, have been used as a treatment option for low HDL "good" cholesterol and high LDL "bad" cholesterol and triglyceride levels.

Used in such large doses, however, nicotinic acid is no longer working as a vitamin, but as a drug, and side effects can occur. Large doses of niacin can cause an increased blood sugar (glucose) level, liver damage, peptic ulcers, and skin rashes.

VITAMIN B5
(Pantothenic Acid)

Pantothenic acid, also known as vitamin B5, is an essential nutrient that is naturally present in some foods, added to other foods, and available as a dietary supplement. The body needs pantothenic acid to convert food into energy and to make red blood cells, certain hormones, and particular fats.

SOURCES OF PANTOTHENIC ACID

Almost all foods contain pantothenic acid in some amount. Pantothenic acid is also added to various foods, including some breakfast cereals and beverages. The best sources include an eclectic mix: eggs, beef, chicken, organ meats, legumes, peanuts, potatoes, avocado, broccoli, mushrooms, milk, whole-grain cereals, and yeast. Fresh vegetables are better sources than canned vegetables because the canning process reduces the amount of pantothenic acid available.

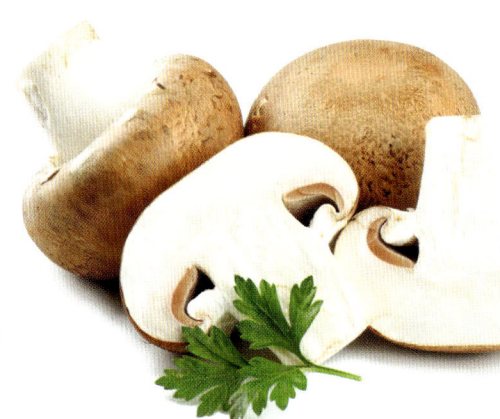

PANTOTHENIC ACID DEFICIENCY

Pantothenic acid deficiency is extremely rare in the United States. Most people get enough pantothenic acid by eating a varied diet. However, people with a rare inherited disorder called pantothenate kinase-associated neurodegeneration can't use pantothenic acid properly. Severe deficiency can cause numbness and burning of hands and feet, headache, extreme fatigue, irritability, restlessness, insomnia, stomach pain, heartburn, diarrhea, nausea, vomiting, and loss of appetite.

VITAMIN B6

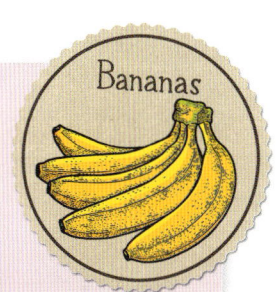
Bananas

Vitamin B6 is the generic name for a group of water-soluble chemical compounds, including pyridoxine, pyridoxal, and pyridoxamine. The body needs vitamin B6 for more than 100 enzyme reactions involved with metabolism.

Researchers discovered early on that vitamin B6 was not one substance but three—pyridoxine, pyridoxal, and pyridoxamine. All three have the same biological activity and all three occur naturally in food. Pyridoxine functions mainly by helping to metabolize protein and amino acids. Though not directly involved in the release of energy, like some other B vitamins, pyridoxine helps remove the nitrogen from amino acids, making them available as sources of energy.

Because of its work with proteins, it plays a role in the synthesis of protein substances such as muscles, antibodies, and hormones. It also helps out in the production of red blood cells, neurotransmitters (chemical messengers), and prostaglandins that regulate certain metabolic processes. This vitamin gets together with more than 60 enzymes in the body, working to get many functions accomplished.

SOURCES OF VITAMIN B6

Vitamin B6 is in all foods, in one form or another. Plant foods are generally high in pyridoxine, while pyridoxamine and pyridoxal are more common in foods of animal origin. All three forms of vitamin B6—pyridoxine, pyridoxamine, and pyridoxal—appear to have the same biological activity.

Protein foods, meats, whole wheat, salmon, nuts, wheat germ, brown rice, peas, and beans are good sources of vitamin B6. Vegetables contain smaller amounts, but if eaten in large quantities, they can be an important source. Even though pyridoxine is lost when grains are milled to make flour, manufacturers do not regularly add it back to enriched products, except some highly fortified cereals.

B6 AND HEALTH

Entire books have been written on the therapeutic uses of vitamin B6; it has been used to treat more than 100 health conditions.

Pyridoxine has a role in preventing heart disease. Without enough pyridoxine, a compound called homocysteine builds up in the body. Homocysteine damages blood vessel linings, setting the stage for plaque buildup when the body tries to heal the damage. Vitamin B6 prevents this buildup, thereby reducing the risk of heart attack. Pyridoxine lowers blood pressure and blood cholesterol levels and keeps blood platelets from sticking together. All of these properties work to keep heart disease at bay.

Prone to kidney stones? Pyridoxine, teamed up with magnesium, prevents the formation of stones. It usually takes about three months of supplementation to make blood levels of these nutrients sufficient to keep stones from forming.

Depression is another condition that may result from low vitamin B6 intake. Because of pyridoxine's role in serotonin and other neurotransmitter production, supplementation often helps depressed people feel better, and their mood improves significantly. It may also help improve memory in older adults. Women who are on hormone-replacement therapy or birth control pills often complain of depression and are frequently deficient in vitamin B6. Supplementation improves these cases, too.

VITAMIN B6 DEFICIENCY AND EXCESS

Most people in the U.S. get enough vitamin B6 from the foods in their diet. However, several groups of people are more likely to have low levels of vitamin B6. These groups include people with kidney problems (such as those who are on kidney dialysis or have had a kidney transplant); people with autoimmune disorders (such as rheumatoid arthritis, celiac disease, Crohn's disease, ulcerative colitis, or inflammatory bowel disease); and people with alcohol dependence.

People with a vitamin B6 deficiency can have a range of symptoms, including anemia, itchy rashes, scaly skin on the lips, cracks at the corners of the mouth, and a swollen tongue. Other symptoms of very low vitamin B6 levels include depression, confusion, and a weak immune system. In infants, vitamin B6 deficiency can cause irritability, extremely sensitive hearing, and seizures.

People almost never get too much vitamin B6 from food sources. However, taking high doses of pyridoxine supplements for an extended period of time can cause severe nerve damage, leading people to lose control of their bodily movements. The symptoms usually disappear when the person stops taking the supplements. Other symptoms of too much vitamin B6 include painful, unsightly skin patches, extreme sensitivity to sunlight, nausea, and heartburn.

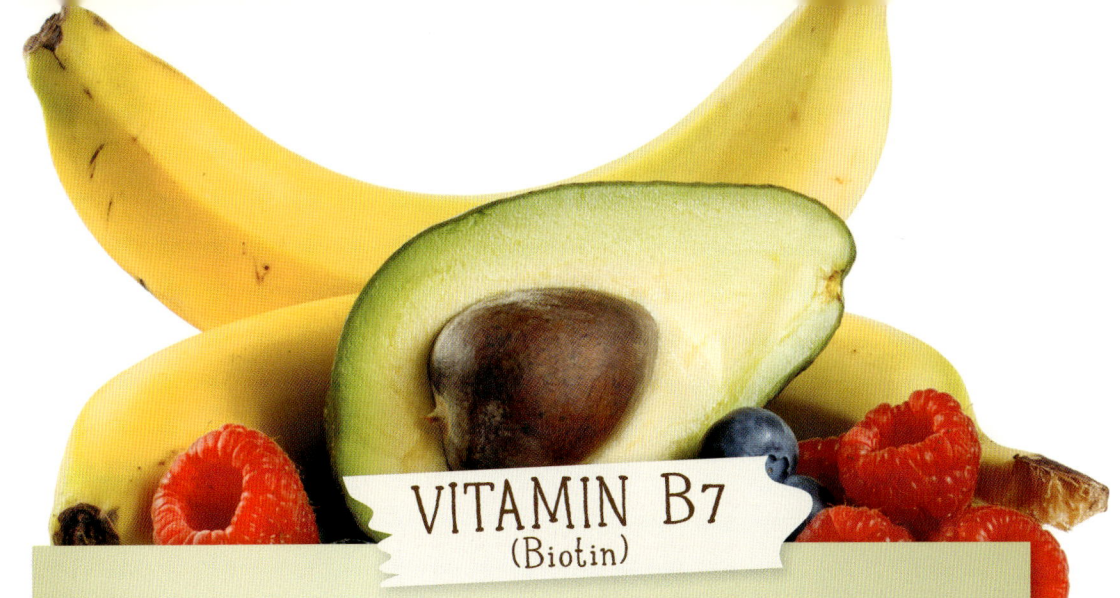

VITAMIN B7
(Biotin)

Biotin is a B vitamin found in many foods, including eggs, meats, and milk. Biotin helps convert the carbohydrates, fats, and proteins in food into energy. Biotin acts as a coenzyme in several metabolic reactions. It plays a role in the manufacture of body fats, the metabolism of carbohydrates, the breakdown of proteins to urea, and the conversion of amino acids from protein into blood sugar for energy.

Mushrooms

SOURCES OF BIOTIN

Milk, liver, eggs, seeds, meats, and fish are sources of biotin. Nuts and mushrooms contain smaller amounts of the vitamin. Bacteria in the intestine also make biotin.

BIOTIN DEFICIENCY

A true biotin deficiency is rare in the United States. However, certain groups of people are more likely to have an inadequate intake of biotin, including people with a rare genetic disorder called biotinidase deficiency, people with alcohol dependence, and women who are pregnant or breastfeeding.

SHOULD YOU SUPPLEMENT?

Biotin supplements may be needed in rare instances. At times, it has been touted as a vitamin that can improve the health of your hair, skin, and nails. But there is little scientific evidence to back up these claims. Biotin can interact with certain medications, and some medications may affect biotin levels. For example, treatment for at least one year with anticonvulsant (antiseizure) medications can significantly lower biotin levels.

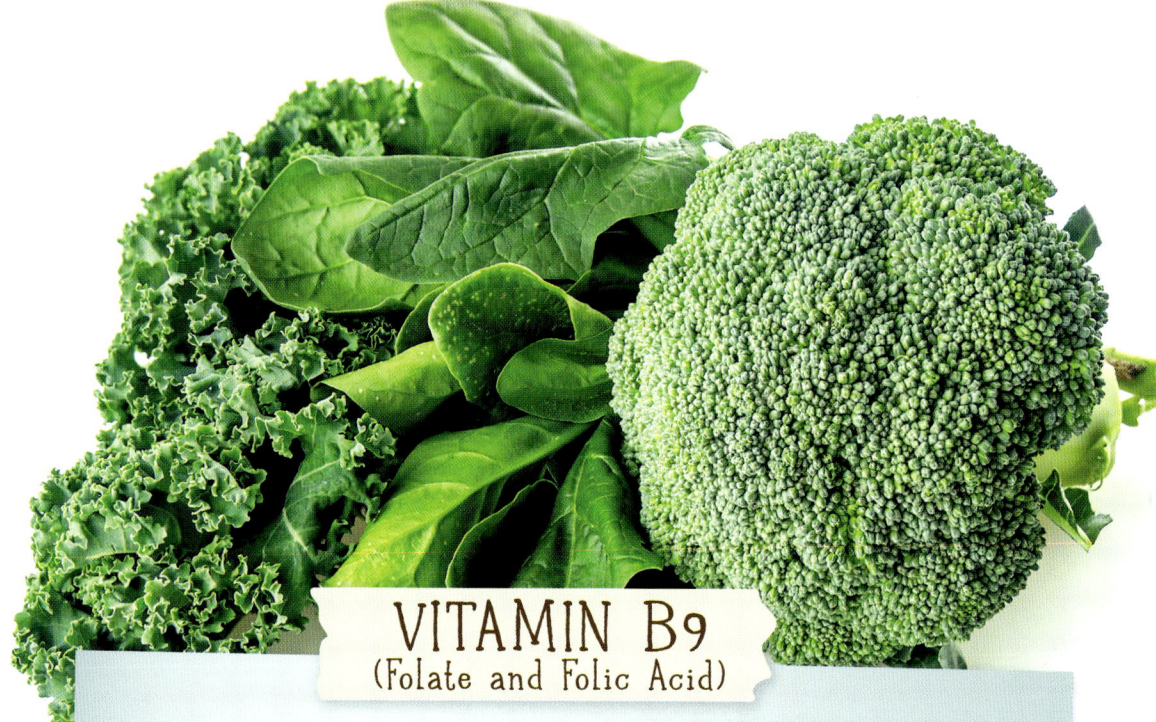

VITAMIN B9
(Folate and Folic Acid)

The discovery of folate was closely tied to the discovery of vitamin B12. These two vitamins work together in several important biological reactions. A deficiency of either vitamin results in a condition known as megaloblastic or macrocytic (large-cell) anemia.

Folate refers to the various forms of the same B vitamin. Folate is naturally present in some foods, added to others, and available as a dietary supplement. Folate occurs naturally in foods such as leafy green vegetables, fruits, and dried beans and peas. Folic acid is the synthetic form of folate used in supplements and fortified foods.

FOLATE AND DNA

Folate functions as a coenzyme during many reactions in the body. It has an important role in making new cells, because it helps form the genetic material DNA (deoxyribonucleic acid) and RNA (ribonucleic acid). DNA carries and RNA transmits the genetic information that acts as the blueprint for cell production.

We especially need folate when new cells are manufactured. This function of folate helps to explain why the vitamin is necessary for normal growth and development, and why anemia occurs when there's not enough. The body makes large numbers of red blood cells each day to replace those it destroys. DNA is essential for this process; therefore, folate is as well.

SOURCES OF FOLATE

Green leafy vegetables, such as broccoli, spinach, and asparagus, are rich in folate. (Take care not to overcook vegetables, or the folate may be lost.) Seeds, liver, and dried peas and beans are other good sources. Orange juice is a good source of folate because it contains the most readily absorbed form of the vitamin. It also contains vitamin C, and vitamin C helps preserve folate.

Folic acid (a form of folate) is available in multivitamins (generally at a dose of 400 mcg) and prenatal vitamins. Folic acid is especially important for women who are pregnant, as it can help prevent major birth defects of the baby's brain or spine. Folic acid is also available in B-complex dietary supplements and found in standalone supplements.

FOLATE DEFICIENCY

Folate deficiency is relatively rare in the United States. Most people get enough folate. However, certain groups are at risk of insufficient folate intakes. These groups include women of childbearing age, non-Hispanic Black women, people with alcohol dependence, and people with disorders that lower nutrient absorption.

Some medications can interfere with the body's ability to use this vitamin. These medications include aspirin, oral contraceptives, and drugs used to treat convulsions, psoriasis, and cancer. In addition, abuse of alcohol can damage the intestine so that less folate is absorbed.

Insufficient folate can result in megaloblastic anemia, which causes weakness, fatigue, trouble concentrating, irritability, headache, heart palpitations, and shortness of breath. Folate deficiency can also cause open sores on the tongue and inside the mouth as well as changes in the color of skin, hair, or fingernails.

Women who don't get enough folate are at risk of having babies with neural tube defects, such as spina bifida. Folate deficiency can also increase the likelihood of having a premature or low-birthweight baby.

Experts now emphasize the importance of folate supplementation in the very early stages of pregnancy because the vitamin plays an important role in early fetal development. Because folate is so important at a time when many women might not even know they are pregnant, women planning to conceive—and any women capable of becoming pregnant—should be sure they are getting enough folate.

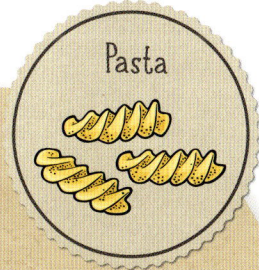

Pasta

FOLIC ACID

Folic acid, the synthetic form of folate, is found in dietary supplements and fortified foods, such as breads, pastas, and cereals.

VITAMIN B12
(Cobalamin)

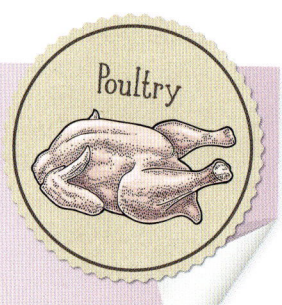
Poultry

Vitamin B12 exists in several forms and contains the mineral cobalt. Vitamin B12 helps maintain healthy nerve and red blood cells, and is needed make DNA (the genetic material in all cells).

INTRINSIC FACTOR

Vitamin B12 differs from other vitamins, even those of the B complex, in many ways. The vitamin has a chemical structure much more complex than that of any other vitamin. It's the only vitamin to contain an inorganic element (cobalt) as an integral part of its makeup. Only microorganisms can make B12. Plants and animals can't, although the vitamin does accumulate in animal products, which is where we get it.

A substance made in the stomach—called intrinsic factor—must be present to absorb vitamin B12 from the intestinal tract in significant amounts. Intrinsic factor combines with the vitamin B12 that is released from food during digestion. It carries the vitamin to the lower part of the small intestine, where, assisted by calcium, it attaches itself to special receptor cells. The vitamin B12 is then released from its carrier and enters these cells to be absorbed into the body. Without intrinsic factor, vitamin B12 misses its connection with the receptor cells and passes out of the body.

People with a condition known as pernicious anemia can't make intrinsic factor. As a result, they can't absorb vitamin B12, even when there's plenty of the vitamin in their diets. Eventually, they show symptoms of a vitamin B12 deficiency. Pernicious anemia is a macrocytic, or large-cell, anemia similar to the anemia caused by folate deficiency.

SOURCES OF B12

Vitamin B12 is naturally found in many animal foods, including beef liver, clams, fish, meat, poultry, eggs, milk, and other dairy products. Manufacturers also add vitamin B12 to some cereals and nutritional yeasts. Plant foods have no vitamin B12 unless they are fortified. Bacteria in the intestines make some vitamin B12, but far less than the amount needed daily.

VITAMIN B12 DEFICIENCY

When the supply of vitamin B12 in the body is low, it slows down the production of red blood cells (causing anemia) and the cells that line the intestine. This is similar to what happens as a result of insufficient folate. But unlike folate deficiency, a lack of vitamin B12 can also cause serious damage to the nervous system. If the condition persists for long, the damage is irreversible.

Most people in the U.S. get enough vitamin B12 from the foods they eat. However, some people have difficulty absorbing vitamin B12 from food. As a result, vitamin B12 deficiency is relatively common, affecting between 1.5 percent and 15 percent of the general public. A deficiency of vitamin B12 caused by insufficient intake is not common. Dietary deficiency of vitamin B12 is usually seen only in strict vegetarians who don't eat foods of animal origin—not even milk or eggs.

VITAMIN C

A major function of vitamin C is its role as a cofactor in the formation and repair of collagen—the connective tissue that holds the body's cells and tissues together. Collagen is a primary component of blood vessels, skin, tendons, and ligaments. Vitamin C also promotes the normal development of bones and teeth. It's also needed for amino acid metabolism and the synthesis of hormones, including the thyroid hormone that controls the body's rate of metabolism. Vitamin C also aids the absorption of iron and calcium.

These days, vitamin C is heralded for its antioxidant status. It prevents other substances from combining with free oxygen radicals by tying up these free radicals of oxygen themselves. In this role, vitamin C protects a number of enzymes involved in functions ranging from cholesterol metabolism to immune function. It destroys harmful free radicals that damage cells and can lead to cancer, heart disease, cataracts, and perhaps even aging. Vitamin C rejuvenates its cousin antioxidant, vitamin E.

SOURCES OF VITAMIN C

Of course, the famed citrus fruits—oranges, lemons, grapefruits, and limes—are excellent sources of vitamin C. Other often overlooked excellent sources of vitamin C are strawberries, kiwifruit, cantaloupe, and peppers. Potatoes also supply vitamin C in significant amounts since they are widely consumed by Americans on a regular basis. Though cooking destroys some of the vitamin, you can minimize the amount lost if the temperature is not too high and you don't cook them any longer than necessary.

For maximum vitamin value, it's best to use fresh, unprocessed fruits and vegetables whenever possible.

Lime

VITAMIN D

Vitamin D is known as the sunshine vitamin for good reason. If you get enough sunshine, your body can make its own vitamin D. Vitamin D (also known as calciferol) is an essential nutrient for building and maintaining strong bones and teeth. It is a unique vitamin—your body can make its own vitamin D when sunlight makes contact with your skin. To get enough, it only takes a few minutes of sun exposure, three times a week, on your hands, arms, or face (without sunscreen). However, if you live in Northern climates or don't get outdoors much, especially in the winter, you shouldn't rely on sunshine. Also, as you age, your body may not be as efficient at making vitamin D, so food sources become even more important.

Vitamin D is necessary to help the body absorb the minerals calcium and phosphorus, which are needed for the proper growth and development of bones and teeth.

Whether it comes from food or is made in the skin, vitamin D must be activated before it's of use to the body. It first travels to the liver, where it undergoes a chemical change. Then it moves through the bloodstream to the kidneys, where it undergoes another change to become the active form of the vitamin. This active form—dihydroxy vitamin D—is the one that helps the body absorb calcium and phosphorus.

Salmon

SOURCES OF VITAMIN D

Your most reliable source of vitamin D is milk. Although milk is fortified with the vitamin, dairy products made from milk such as cheese, yogurt, and ice cream are generally not fortified with vitamin D. Only a few foods, including fatty fish (such as salmon, tuna, and mackerel) and fish oils, naturally contain significant amounts of vitamin D.

Other foods that contain smaller amounts of vitamin D include eggs, margarine, beef liver, and mushrooms, as well as fortified breakfast cereals, orange juice, yogurt, margarine, and soy beverages. The vitamin D in supplements and fortified foods is found in two different forms: D2 (ergocalciferol) and D3 (cholecalciferol). Both increase vitamin D in the blood.

VITAMIN D DEFICIENCY

People can become vitamin D deficient because they don't consume or absorb enough from food, their sunlight exposure is limited, or their kidneys cannot convert vitamin D to its active form in the body. In children, vitamin D deficiency causes rickets. Though rickets is rare in the United States today, some cases still occur, especially among African American infants and children. Vitamin D deficiency in adults leads to osteomalacia, which causes bone pain and muscle weakness.

TOXICITY

Too much vitamin D can actually be toxic, especially to children. Symptoms of overdose include diarrhea, nausea, vomiting, headache, weakness, weight loss, and elevated calcium levels in the blood.

VITAMIN E

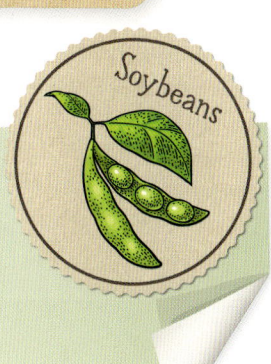

Soybeans

Vitamin E is not a single compound, but several different compounds, all with vitamin E activity. One, alpha-tocopherol (or α-tocopherol), has the greatest activity. Other compounds with vitamin E activity are beta-tocopherol, gamma-tocopherol, and delta-tocopherol.

FUNCTIONS OF VITAMIN E

Vitamin E functions as an antioxidant in the cells and tissues of the body. It protects polyunsaturated fats and other oxygen-sensitive compounds such as vitamin A from being destroyed by damaging oxidation reactions.

Vitamin E's antioxidant properties are also important to cell membranes. For example, vitamin E protects lung cells that are in constant contact with oxygen and white blood cells that help fight disease. A deficiency of vitamin E thus weakens the immune system. But the benefits of vitamin E's antioxidant role may go much further. Vitamin E may protect against heart disease and may slow the deterioration associated with aging. Critics scoffed at such claims in the past, but an understanding of the importance of vitamin E's antioxidant role may be beginning to pay off.

SOURCES OF VITAMIN E

Oils and margarines from corn, cottonseed, soybean, safflower, and wheat germ are all good sources of vitamin E. Generally, the more polyunsaturated oil is, the more vitamin E it contains, serving as its own built-in protection. Fruits, vegetables, and whole grains have smaller amounts. Refining grains reduces their vitamin E content, as does commercial processing and storage of food. Cooking foods at high temperatures also destroys vitamin E, so a polyunsaturated oil is useless as a vitamin E source if it's used for frying. Your best sources are fresh and lightly processed foods, as well as those that aren't overcooked.

VITAMIN K

Broccoli

Vitamin K is the generic name for a family of compounds with a common chemical structure. These include phylloquinone (vitamin K1), menaquinone (vitamin K2), and menadione (vitamin K3). Vitamin K plays an important role in forming blood clots and maintaining strong bones, and also has other functions in the body. The proteins used in blood clotting require vitamin K. When there isn't enough of the vitamin, blood takes longer to clot, which can increase the amount of blood lost. Vitamin K also helps make a protein that may help regulate blood calcium levels. Calcium, usually associated with keeping bones strong, is also necessary for blood clotting.

SOURCES OF VITAMIN K

Food sources of vitamin K include green leafy vegetables (such as kale, spinach, broccoli, and lettuce), vegetable oils (such as soybean and canola oil), some fruits (such as blueberries and figs), meat, cheese, eggs, and soybeans. The best food sources of phylloquinone (vitamin K1) are green leafy vegetables (especially collards, turnip greens, spinach, kale, parsley, and broccoli), pumpkin, okra, soybean oil, carrot juice, pomegranate juice, and prunes. Meat, dairy products, and eggs contain low levels of phylloquinone but modest amounts of menaquinone (vitamin K2).

We get some of the vitamin K we need from the foods we eat. The rest comes from the bacteria that live in our digestive tracts and produce vitamin K. The extent to which we are able to use bacterially produced vitamin K, however, is still somewhat uncertain.

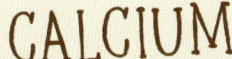

CALCIUM

Building strong bones and teeth is the most familiar function of calcium. Indeed, those bones and teeth contain 99 percent of all the calcium in your body. The remaining one percent circulates in blood or resides in the body's soft tissues. This one percent, however, plays many extremely important roles. It participates in blood clotting, contraction and relaxation of muscles, transmission of nerve impulses, activation of enzymes, and hormone secretion.

Because maintaining a normal blood calcium level is so important to vital functions such as heart rhythm, the body has a way to ensure a constant level of calcium in the blood, no matter how much your diet provides. The secret reservoir of calcium happens to be your bones, which release calcium into the blood as needed. But if this happens too rapidly, your bones suffer the consequences.

SOURCES OF CALCIUM

Milk, yogurt, cheese, and other dairy products are rich sources of calcium. Dried beans and peas and green vegetables such as broccoli, kale, bok choy, and chard are also good sources.

Phytic acid, a substance found in whole grains, can reduce calcium absorption. Oxalic acid, which is found in some vegetables and beans, can also reduce calcium absorption. Vitamin D increases calcium absorption.

CALCIUM DEFICIENCY

A deficiency of calcium can stunt the development of bones and teeth. A lack of vitamin D, which is needed for calcium's absorption and use, can have a similar effect. Bones suffer the brunt of insufficient calcium because they defer their needs to other functions that demand a higher priority. Blood clotting and muscle contraction are critical functions of calcium that must be sustained to preserve life. If muscle contractions go awry, your heart can stop. So when the blood contains too little calcium, bones give up their calcium for these functions. If this happens too often, bones become porous and weak.

The result of such weakening is osteoporosis. Osteoporosis is a condition in which bones become porous, fragile, and prone to fracture.

CHLORINE

Chlorine is an important regulator of body systems, such as water balance, acid-base balance, and fluid pressure. For example, this mineral is part of hydrochloric acid, needed in the stomach for digestion. The acidity it creates ensures proper absorption of food and reduces the growth of harmful bacteria.

There is no recommended daily allowance for chlorine. Regular table salt is 60 percent chlorine, as chloride. This source, along with the salt that occurs naturally in foods, provides all the chlorine that's needed. Even a diet restricted in sodium can supply adequate amounts of chlorine.

Shrimp

CHROMIUM

Chromium is part of the glucose tolerance factor (GTF) that regulates the actions of insulin—the hormone necessary for glucose metabolism. In chromium-deficient people, insulin doesn't function properly. In such cases, chromium supplements can improve the body's ability to handle glucose. Chromium is also important in the metabolism of fats and carbohydrates.

SOURCES OF CHROMIUM

Chromium is an essential mineral not made by the body—it must be obtained from the diet. A diet rich in refined carbohydrates such as sugar increases the need for chromium. And the more refined and processed foods are, the less chromium they contain.

Brewer's yeast and wheat germ are rich in chromium. Other sources include whole grains, meats, poultry, cheese and other dairy products, seafood, broccoli, and eggs.

COBALT

Cobalt is needed in very small amounts. As part of vitamin B12, cobalt plays a major role in the body's metabolic processes. There is no RDA for cobalt because it is usually obtained from vitamin B12. A cobalt deficiency can lead to anemia. Too much cobalt can lead to a greater than normal number of red blood cells.

COPPER

Copper helps the body absorb and use iron. It's part of several enzymes that help form hemoglobin (the oxygen-carrying pigment in red blood cells) and collagen (a connective-tissue protein found in skin and tendons). Copper also helps keep the immune system, blood vessels, nerves, and bones healthy.

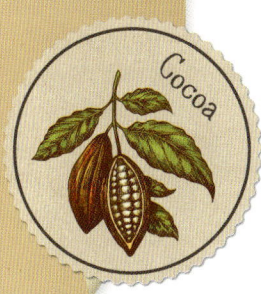
Cocoa

SOURCES OF COPPER

Good sources of copper include oysters and other shellfish, whole grains, potatoes, beans, nuts, and liver. Prunes and other dried fruits, dark leafy greens, cocoa, yeast, and black pepper are also decent sources of copper.

FLUORIDE

Fluoride is an essential trace mineral found in bones, teeth, and body fluids. If fluoride is available when bones and teeth develop, it's incorporated into their structures, making teeth more resistant to decay and bones more resistant to osteoporosis. Fluoride also maintains the structure of bones and teeth after they are formed.

SOURCES OF FLUORIDE

Water is the most common source of fluoride in the diet. Food prepared in fluoridated water also contains fluoride. Most seafood contains fluoride since there is natural sodium fluoride in the ocean. Tea is a surprisingly good source as well. A cup of tea provides about 0.2 milligrams of fluoride.

Research shows that people who live in areas where the drinking water contains less than one part per million of fluoride have more dental decay and osteoporosis.

IODINE

Iodine is a trace element naturally present in some foods, added to others, and available in the form of supplements. Iodine is an important component of thyroid hormones, which control energy metabolism in the body. Thyroid hormones are also required for proper bone and brain development during pregnancy and infancy.

SOURCES OF IODINE

Saltwater seafood is a primary source of iodine. Iodized salt, in use since 1924, is another rich source. One teaspoon of iodized salt provides 260 micrograms (mcg) of iodine. The amount of iodine in vegetables and grains varies according to how much is present in the soil where they are grown. In certain regions of the world, this amount is less than optimal.

In the United States, the need for iodized salt is not as great as it was 60 years ago. Thanks to refrigerated trucks, most of the country gets produce from coastal regions where soil is rich in iodine. Iodine deficiency is a concern only in isolated areas where all the food eaten is locally grown.

IODINE DEFICIENCY

A deficiency of iodine can cause the thyroid gland to greatly enlarge—a condition known as goiter. The thyroid gland, which is normally about the size of a lima bean, can sometimes become as large as a person's head. A deficiency of thyroid hormones can result in mental and physical sluggishness, slowed heart rate, weight gain, constipation, and increased sleep needs (14–16 hours a day). In pregnancy, the results of iodine deficiency are more serious.

Substances known as goitrogens induce goiter when iodine intake is low. Cabbage, Brussels sprouts, cauliflower, turnips, and peanuts contain these substances. However, since heat destroys goitrogens, the potential dangers exist only if large amounts of these foods are eaten raw.

IRON

Most of the body's iron resides in the hemoglobin of red blood cells—the pigment that makes these blood cells appear red. Hemoglobin carries oxygen to cells and transports carbon dioxide from cells. Iron is also essential to enzymes involved in energy release, cholesterol metabolism, immune function, and connective-tissue production.

SOURCES OF IRON

Iron in food comes in two forms—heme iron and nonheme iron. Lean meat and seafood are the richest dietary sources of heme iron. Sources of nonheme iron include nuts, beans, vegetables, and fortified grain products. Meat, seafood, and poultry have both heme and nonheme iron.

Other food sources of iron include white beans, lentils, spinach, kidney beans, peas, dark chocolate, tofu, and raisins. Nonheme iron from plant sources is better absorbed when eaten with meat, poultry, seafood, and vitamin C-rich foods (e.g., citrus fruits, strawberries, sweet peppers, tomatoes, and broccoli).

IRON DEFICIENCY

Iron deficiency anemia may not cause obvious symptoms at first. But as the body uses its stored iron and the anemia worsens, the signs and symptoms intensify. Tiredness and lack of energy; chest pain, heart palpitations, or shortness of breath; headache, dizziness, or lightheadedness; poor memory and concentration; and sore tongue are some of the symptoms of iron deficiency anemia. For people who are anemic, even mild exercise can cause chest pain.

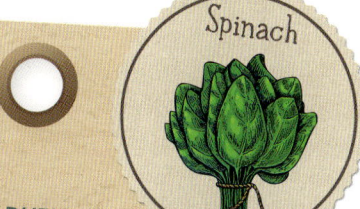

Spinach

A SERIOUS WARNING

Iron poisoning is the most common accidental poisoning in young children. Excess iron can be fatal. All supplements should be kept out of the reach of children.

MAGNESIUM

Magnesium is a mineral the body needs for healthy nerves, muscles, and bones. Magnesium is a vital part of the mineral structure of bones and teeth. As with calcium, bones act as a reservoir for magnesium so that it will be available when needed.

Magnesium plays a role in protein synthesis, muscle relaxation, and energy release. It also triggers important metabolic reactions, including calcium metabolism. The parathyroid hormone needs magnesium to function normally; this regulates blood calcium levels.

SOURCES OF MAGNESIUM

Magnesium is found in many foods, particularly green leafy vegetables. This is because magnesium is part of chlorophyll, the pigment in plants that makes them green and fosters photosynthesis. Some breakfast cereals are fortified with magnesium. Other sources of magnesium are nuts and seeds; peas and beans; dairy products; whole grains; and chocolate. Hard water also contains significant amounts of magnesium.

MAGNESIUM DEFICIENCY

Nutritional surveys show that most people in the United States get less than the recommended amounts of magnesium from food. Men over 70 and adolescent girls are the most likely to have low magnesium intakes. However, when magnesium from food and supplements are combined, the total intakes are usually above recommended amounts.

Loss of appetite, vomiting, nausea, fatigue, and weakness are early signs of magnesium deficiency. As the condition worsens, magnesium deficiency can cause numbness, tingling, muscle cramps, seizures, personality changes, and abnormal heart rhythms.

MAGNESIUM TOXICITY

High intakes of magnesium from food are rarely a concern for healthy people since the kidneys eliminate excess amounts in urine. However, high doses of magnesium from dietary supplements can cause diarrhea, nausea, and abdominal cramps.

MANGANESE

Manganese is a mineral that helps ensure proper bone formation and connective-tissue growth. It activates many enzymes that regulate metabolism. It may also play a role as an antioxidant, as part of the enzyme superoxide dismutase.

SOURCES OF MANGANESE

Good sources of manganese include nuts, seeds, legumes, whole grains, tea, and leafy greens. Manganese is also available in dietary supplements. It is frequently included in supplements for osteoarthritis.

TOO MUCH

Too much manganese can cause unwanted side effects. People with liver disease and those with iron deficiency anemia should be especially careful not to get too much manganese.

MOLYBDENUM

This hard-to-pronounce mineral (muh LIB duh num) functions as part of the enzyme systems involved in carbohydrate, fat, and protein metabolism. Humans need only very small amounts of molybdenum, which are easily acquired through a healthy diet.

SOURCES OF MOLYBDENUM

Good sources of molybdenum are liver, wheat germ, whole grains, nuts, and legumes. The molybdenum content of food varies according to what was in the soil from which it came.

PHOSPHORUS

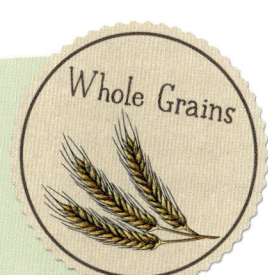

Whole Grains

Phosphorus is a mineral that is vital for strong bones and teeth. Phosphorus also plays an important role in energy storage and release. It's found in DNA (deoxyribonucleic acid) and RNA (ribonucleic acid), the genetic materials that serve as the blueprints for the formation of new cells. Phosphorus is necessary for normal milk secretion and a variety of metabolic reactions as well.

SOURCES OF PHOSPHORUS

Good sources of phosphorus are also good sources of protein—for example, such foods as milk and other dairy products, eggs, meat, fish, poultry, nuts, and whole grains are good sources of both. Fruits and vegetables contain only small amounts of phosphorus. Phosphorus is added to many processed foods. Even sodas and food additives supply some phosphorus. As a result, most Americans get plenty of phosphorus from their diet.

PROTEIN AND PHOSPHORUS

Americans consume as much as four times their recommended daily allowance of phosphorus. American diets are heavy in high-protein foods (such as meat, fish, or poultry), carbonated beverages, and ready-to-eat convenience foods—all of which increase the body's supply of phosphorus. However, phosphorus deficiency has been reported in some infants fed cow's milk and in some people taking large amounts of antacids.

POTASSIUM

Potassium is a mineral that the body needs for cells, nerves, and muscles to function properly. Potassium plays an important role in maintaining water balance and acid-base balance. Its presence is crucial in the transmission of nerve impulses from nerves to muscles. It also acts as a catalyst in carbohydrate and protein metabolism.

SOURCES OF POTASSIUM

While almost all whole foods contain some potassium, particularly good sources include apricots, prunes, legumes, squash, potatoes, milk, tomatoes, bananas, oranges, and meat. Fruits and vegetables reign supreme in the potassium-supply category. Processed foods, on the other hand, lose much of their potassium during processing.

POTASSIUM DEFICIENCY AND EXCESS

Having too much or too little potassium in the body can cause serious health problems. A low level of potassium is called hypokalemia. A high level of potassium in the blood is called hyperkalemia. Dietary surveys consistently show that most people in the United States consume much less potassium than recommended. Not getting enough potassium can increase blood pressure, deplete calcium in bones, and increase the risk of kidney stones.

Hypokalemia can be caused by certain kidney or adrenal gland disorders, prolonged vomiting and diarrhea, laxative abuse, use of diuretics, excessive sweating, and dialysis. Symptoms of hypokalemia include constipation, tiredness, muscle weakness, increased urination, decreased brain function, high blood sugar levels, muscle paralysis, difficulty breathing, and irregular heartbeat.

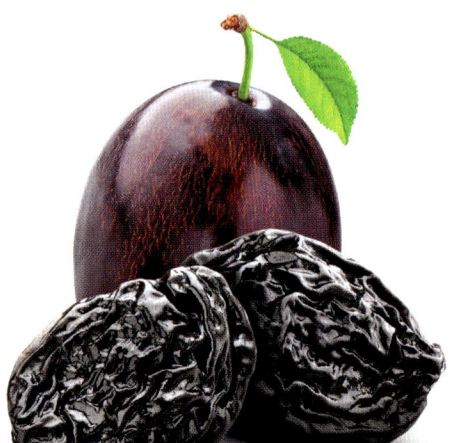

SALT SUBSTITUTES

Potassium combined with chloride is effective at restoring potassium losses from the body and can satisfy a taste for table salt. In fact, many salt substitutes are compounds of potassium chloride. People with kidney disease, however, should avoid them.

SELENIUM

Selenium is a mineral important for reproduction, thyroid gland function, DNA production, and protecting the body from free radical damage and infection.

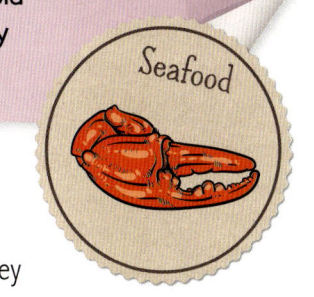
Seafood

SOURCES OF SELENIUM

Selenium is naturally present in many foods. The amount of selenium in plant foods depends on the selenium content of the soil in which they were grown. For animal products, the amount depends on the selenium content of the foods the animals ate.

A super source of selenium is the Brazil nut, with 68–91 micrograms (mcg) per nut. Seafood and organ meats are also rich in selenium. Other food sources include poultry, eggs, dairy products, breads, cereals, and other grain products. The daily value (DV) for selenium is 70 micrograms for adults and children over age 4.

SODIUM

Sodium plays a critical role in regulating water balance in the body. It's also important for regulating acid-base balance, transmitting nerve impulses, maintaining muscle activity and cell membrane function, and absorbing and transporting certain nutrients. Sodium is also a part of body fluids such as sweat and tears.

SOURCES OF SODIUM

The majority of sodium in the typical American diet comes from processed and prepared foods. Processed foods include bread, crackers, breakfast cereals, pizza, microwavable dinners, canned vegetables, soups, sauces, deli meat, cheese, fast foods, and prepared dinners such as pasta, meat, and egg dishes. Sodium is naturally present in some foods, including vegetables, dairy products, meat, and shellfish. Celery, carrots, artichokes, beets, eggs, and milk are naturally high in sodium. Another source of sodium is the salt used in cooking or at the table.

TOO MUCH OR TOO LITTLE

On average, Americans consume more than 3,400 milligrams of sodium per day. This far exceeds what the body actually needs to function properly. Current recommendations suggest limiting sodium to less than 2,300 milligrams per day. Certain groups, including adults with prehypertension and hypertension, should limit intake to 1,500 milligrams per day. Sodium sensitive people should also further limit sodium intake. Sodium sensitive people retain sodium more easily, leading to fluid retention and increased blood pressure (hypertension).

Excessive intake of sodium is a much more common problem than deficiency. Consuming too much sodium puts you at risk for developing serious medical conditions like high blood pressure (hypertension), heart disease, and stroke.

Because the body has a large sodium reserve and, under normal circumstances, people eat plenty of sodium-containing foods, a deficiency is not likely. However, salt depletion can temporarily occur through profuse sweating if you exercise strenuously for a prolonged time in warm weather or hot climates. Even in this situation, salt that's lost is easily replaced.

SULFUR

Sulfur is found throughout the body, especially in the skin, hair, and nails. The mineral aids in the storage and release of energy. It's a component of the genetic material of cells, and it helps promote enzyme reactions and blood clotting. Sulfur is part of two B vitamins—biotin and thiamin. Sulfur also combines with certain toxic materials so they can then be excreted safely from the body through the urine.

SOURCES OF SULFUR

A wide variety of foods contain sulfur. Cheese, eggs, fish, poultry, grains, nuts, and dried peas and beans are all rich sources.

When protein intake is adequate, sulfur intake is adequate as well. That's because sulfur-containing amino acids (the building blocks of protein) supply the body with the amount of sulfur it needs. However, getting adequate amounts of sulfur from other sources preserves these amino acids for their other vital functions.

ZINC

Most zinc resides in our bones. The rest of this trace mineral turns up in skin, hair, and nails. In men, the prostate gland contains more zinc than any other organ. Zinc is a part of more than 200 different enzyme systems that aid the metabolism of carbohydrates, fats, and proteins. One of these enzymes, superoxide dismutase, serves as an antioxidant in cells. Zinc is also part of the hormone insulin, helping transport vitamin A from its storage site in the liver to where it is used in the body.

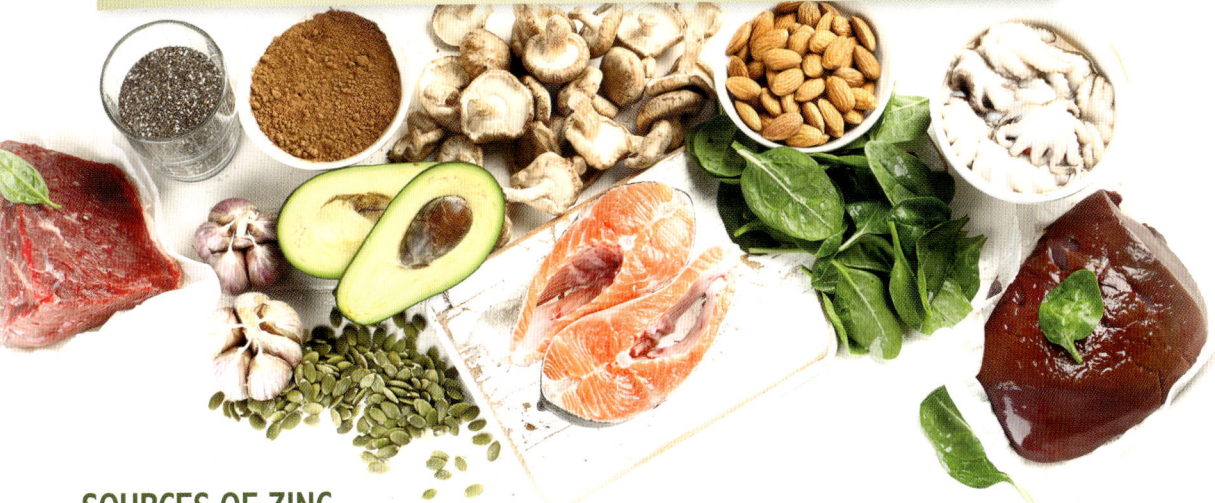

SOURCES OF ZINC

Oysters contain more zinc than any other food. Meat, poultry, seafood, eggs, liver, and fortified breakfast cereals are also rich sources. Beans, nuts, dairy products, and whole grains provide some zinc. Two servings of animal protein daily provide most of the zinc a healthy person needs. Whole grains contain fair amounts of zinc, but they also harbor phytates, substances that tie up zinc and other minerals and prevent absorption. Yeast counteracts the action of phytates, so eating whole-grain breads still affords good nutrition.

ZINC AND THE IMMUNE SYSTEM

Optimal immune function is vital for avoiding colds, flu, cancer, and infectious diseases in general. Zinc supplements before and during an illness can help the body put up a better fight. Zinc lozenges dissolved slowly in the mouth help to resolve a cold and sore throat. Viruses responsible for illness are inhibited by zinc; they're unable to replicate.

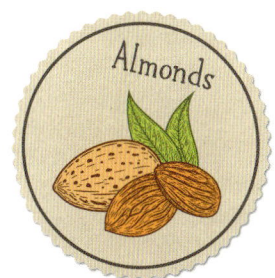

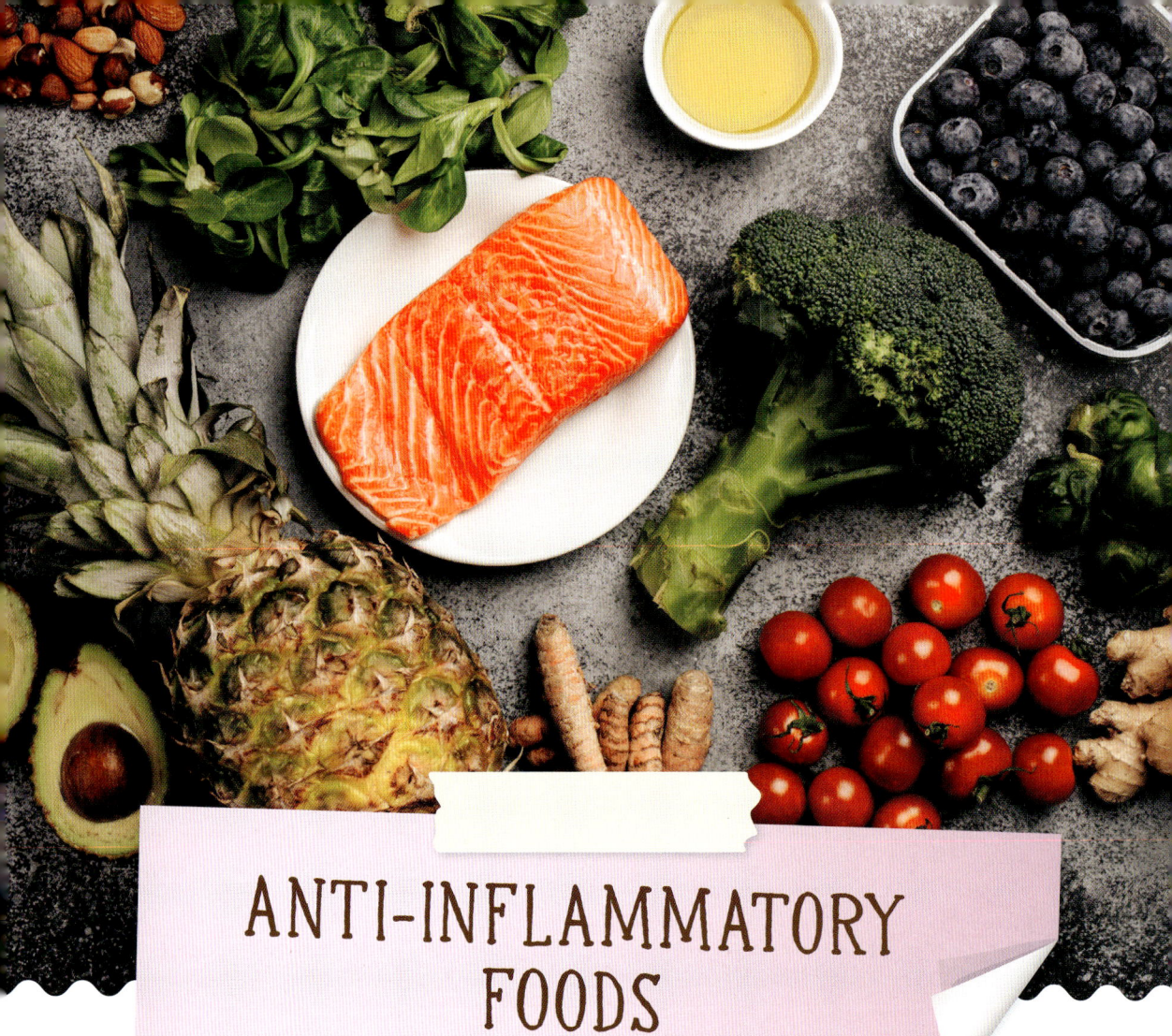

ANTI-INFLAMMATORY FOODS

A painful cut that puffs and reddens. A skinned knee that is sore to the touch. A reddened eye that itches and tears. These conditions may signify acute inflammation, a complex biological response to what the body perceives as potentially harmful injury or stimuli.

Unending stomach or intestinal cramps and discomfort. Constant joint and muscular aches and pains. Lingering sinusitis and allergic-type symptoms. These conditions may signal chronic inflammation, a complex biological response to longer-term "wear and tear" on the body with multiple causes and outcomes. Some have speculated that what you eat can affect your levels of chronic inflammation and thus your overall comfort and health.

Acute Inflammation

Acute inflammation is the early and sometimes immediate response by the human body to potentially harmful bacteria or an injury to bodily tissues. In acute inflammation, damaged cells, foreign invaders such as bacteria and viruses, irritants, and pathogens, bombard the body and activate blood vessels, immune cells, and molecular modulators to respond and repair.

The onset of acute inflammation may last just a few days and it generally improves on its own. Acute appendicitis, bronchitis, infected ingrown nails, infective meningitis, physical trauma, sinusitis, skin abrasions, sore throat from cold or flu, or tonsillitis may trigger acute inflammation.

IN THE LONG TERM

If acute inflammation lasts longer and if the inflamed site becomes abscessed, then this may mark infection or a longer, more chronic condition.

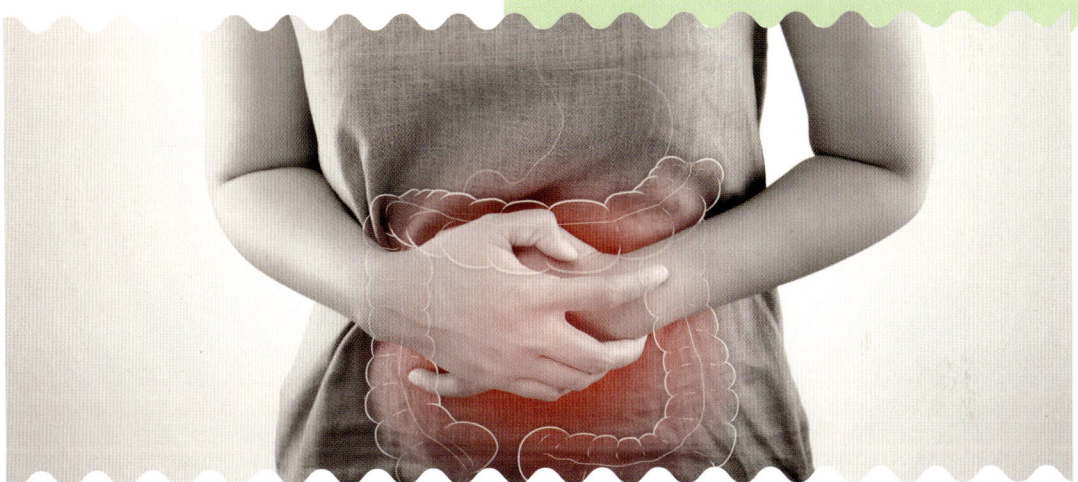

Chronic Inflammation

Chronic inflammation is typically longer in duration than acute inflammation and due more to "use and abuse" than acute injuries. Chronic inflammation may be initiated by pathogens that the body has a difficult time destroying. It may not be as noticeable as acute inflammation—especially if sensory nerve endings are not close enough to affected areas to register pain. The onset may be slow, starting from days and lasting from months to years. Symptoms of chronic inflammation may include abdominal, chest, joint and muscular pain; fatigue; fever; mouth sores; and rashes.

Factors that contribute to chronic inflammation may include alcohol ingestion, diet, drug use, environmental conditions, genes, inactivity, oral health, smoking, stress, weight, and autoimmune diseases.

Autoimmune diseases are illnesses that occur when body tissues are attacked by the immune system. For example, lupus and rheumatoid arthritis may have inflammatory origins, as well as pernicious anemia and Type 1 diabetes. Conditions and diseases that may be caused by chronic inflammation may include active hepatitis, arthritis (gouty, osteo-, psoriatic, and rheumatoid), asthma, Crohn's disease, chronic peptic ulcer, diverticula disease, fibromyalgia, periodontitis, sinusitis, tuberculosis, ulcerative colitis, and more.

Chronic inflammation may lead to thickening and scaring of connective tissues and even tissue death. Longer term, untreated chronic inflammation may cause more complicated health problems, such as atherosclerosis, bone disease, diabetes, hypertension, and some cancers.

Immune Health

Since inflammation has both acute and chronic expressions, it is difficult to pinpoint their relationship to immune health. Some generic factors may also come into play. People with healthy immune systems are generally able to defend themselves against some shorter and longer-term inflammatory conditions or diseases. They may have acquired "adaptive" immunity that developed after an infection or vaccination, inherited a healthy immune system, taken excellent care of their health, been lucky, or benefitted by many of these factors.

Identification, Treatment, and Control

Now that we know more about what inflammation is, let's talk about how to recognize and reduce it. Diet, exercise, and medication can all play a role.

IDENTIFICATION

Acute inflammatory disease may be identified by an abrasion, contusion, redness, or swelling. Chronic inflammation may be more complicated to identify; therefore blood tests, medical histories, physical exams, X-rays, or other electronic procedures may be necessary.

For example, C-reactive protein (CRP) is a blood test marker for infection or inflammation. The liver produces C-reactive protein that rises in response to inflammation. A CRP level over 3.0 mg/dL may pose a higher-than-normal risk of certain chronic diseases such as cardiovascular disease.

TREATMENT

Acute inflammation is typically treated with topical analgesics and other over-the-counter medications unless it persists and becomes infected. Then, medical attention is advised.

Controlling chronic inflammation often involves a combination of treatment approaches. These may include behavior modification, diet, exercise, medications, physical therapy, rest or sleep, yoga, or surgery in some cases. Efforts should be taken to avoid or modify activities that aggravate or induce the most pain.

Many drugs may help decrease joint pain, inflammation, overall discomfort and swelling—independently or in combination with others. The use of drugs or herbs to relieve inflammation should be under the guidance of health care professionals.

CONTROL: DIET AND NUTRITION

One of the most important and often overlooked methods of prevention, treatment, and control of inflammation is diet and nutrition. The building blocks of a nutritious diet are the carbohydrates, fats, proteins, vitamins, and minerals that are found in a variety of lean proteins, lower-fat dairy products, fresh fruits and vegetables, healthy fats, nuts and seeds, and whole grains. They provide the foundation of anti-inflammatory eating.

Other substances such as chocolate, coffee and tea, fermented foods, herbs and spices, and pre- and probiotics, along with adequate hydration and supplements, if needed, round out a spectrum of anti-inflammatory measures.

Hard evidence for one type of anti-inflammatory method over another may be lacking, but collectively some of these approaches may be effective. It is best to check any dietary approaches with a health care provider.

> **NATURAL REMEDIES**
>
> Cannabis, ginger, and turmeric are some of the herbal remedies that may also be used to treat various types of inflammation.

Use, Limit, Avoid

An anti-inflammatory approach to diet and nutrition is mostly founded on a Mediterranean-type diet that emphasizes the following foods with fiber-rich carbohydrates, lean proteins, healthy fats, and disease-fighting vitamins and minerals:

- **Cold-water fish** (herring, mackerel, salmon, sardines, and tuna) with omega 3-fatty acids.
- **Fresh fruits and vegetables** (berries, oranges, broccoli, and cauliflower) with plant-based phytonutrients (antioxidants, flavonoids, and plant sterols).

- **Nuts and seeds and their oils** (almonds and walnuts) with heart-healthy monounsaturated fatty acids and vitamin E.
- **Whole grains** (quinoa and steel-cut oats) with hearty fibers for cardiovascular and digestive health and calorie control.

CARBOHYDRATES

Carbohydrates provide calories in the forms of starches and sugars that convert into glucose, the body's main dietary source of energy. Carbohydrates vary significantly in their nutritional benefits and relationship to chronic inflammation. They are often classified as high-glycemic (HG) carbohydrates and low-glycemic (HG) carbohydrates according to how fast they convert into glucose and affect blood sugar levels.

High-glycemic (HG) carbohydrates typically have more impact on blood sugar. HG-carbohydrates include cakes, candies, cookies, soft drinks, and processed foods made with white flours. HG-carbohydrates have been connected with increased levels of C-reactive protein, may trigger or worsen chronic inflammation, and add calories.

Low-glycemic (LG) carbohydrates tend to digest slowly and generally have less impact on blood sugar. LG-carbohydrates include fresh fruits and vegetables, legumes (dried beans, lentils, and peas), unsweetened dairy products, and whole grains. LG-carbohydrates may also help to reduce or stabilize chronic inflammation.

Use: In general, replace refined HG-carbohydrates with unrefined LG-carbohydrates that provide more antioxidants, fibers, protein, vitamins, and minerals for improved blood sugar control and less chronic inflammation.

Limit: Natural sugars, such as agave, honey, maple syrup, and molasses with some trace micronutrients. Non-caloric artificial sweeteners (NAS), such as aspartame (Equal), saccharine (Sweet 'n Low), and sucralose (Splenda) may alter GI bacteria and affect how the body handles glucose.

Avoid: Refined grains made with processed white flours. Sugars, since they tend to spike blood sugar levels and contain more calories than nutrients.

GRAINY GOODNESS

Whole grains include amaranth, barley, bulgur, einkorn, emmer, farro, kamut, millet, oats (especially steel cut), rye, spelt, teff, triticale, and wheat berries. Some whole grains are considered "ancient grains" which mean they have not been modified or crossbred throughout the years. Buckwheat groats (kasha), quinoa, and basmati, brown and wild rice are technically seeds, though often grouped as whole grains, like couscous that is tiny pasta.

 Food Pharmacy

Sugars include those with the suffix "-ose" (such as dextrose, galactose, glucose, lactose, and maltose), as well as barley malt, beet sugar, brown sugar, buttered syrup, cane juice, date sugar, dehydrated cane juice, cane juice solids, cane juice crystals, caramel, carob crystals, carob syrup, corn syrup, corn syrup solids, dehydrated fruit juice, date sugar, diatase, diatastic malt, dextrin, dextran, ethyl maltol, fruit juice, fruit juice concentrate, fruit juice crystals, golden syrup, honey, maltodextrin, malt syrup, maple syrup, Refiner's syrup, sorghum syrup, turbinado sugar, yellow sugar, and others, should also be avoided.

FRUITS

Whole seasonable fresh fruits are preferred for their rich sources of antioxidant and anti-inflammatory carotenoids and flavonoids.

Use: The best anti-inflammatory fruit choices include apples, apricots, bananas, blueberries, blackberries, cherries, cranberries, fresh figs, kiwi, melons, nectarines, oranges, peaches, pears, pink grapefruit, plums, pomegranates, red grapes, and strawberries. Berries contain anthocyanins, polyphenol compounds that may moderate inflammation. Cherries contain analgesic substances and anthocyanins. Citrus fruits such as grapefruits, lemons, limes, and oranges contain antioxidant vitamin C and flavonoids that may neutralize free radicals.

Limit: Canned or frozen fruits in fruit juice. Additionally, citrus fruits may be limited for people with citrus sensitivities since they may contribute to inflammation under certain conditions.

Avoid: Canned or frozen fruits in sugar syrup, dried fruits, and fruit juices packed with added sugars.

> **AWESOME APPLES**
>
> An apple a day may not keep the doctor away, but apples are high in insoluble and soluble fibers (pectin) that may curb appetite, antioxidant vitamins A and C, and polyphenols that may lower levels of cholesterol and C-reactive protein.

VEGETABLES

Fresh and lightly cooked vegetables are recommended for their antioxidant and anti-inflammatory carotenoids and flavonoids.

Use: Emphasize these vegetables with their noteworthy anti-inflammatory substances: garlic, onions, broccoli and crucifers, fermented probiotic vegetables (kimchi, pickles, and sauerkraut), romaine lettuce, spinach, and Swiss chard. Sea vegetables (edible seaweed) such as arame, brown algae, dulse, kelp, nori, and wakame contain antioxidant carotenoids and polyphenols and may block pro-inflammatory cytokines and other potentially inflammatory substances. Mushrooms (fungi) such as organic enokitake, maitake, and oyster mushrooms contain antioxidants that may have anti-cancer, anti-inflammatory, and immune-enhancing effects.

Limit: Nightshade vegetables (bell peppers, chilies, eggplant, potatoes, and tomatoes) that contain glycoalkaloids, and natural pesticides associated with some arthritic symptoms that include joint pain. However, some nightshade vegetables contain appreciable amounts of antioxidant vitamins A and C that may combat inflammation.

Avoid: Breaded, fried, salted, or sauced vegetables that are higher in calories, refined carbohydrates, sodium, and sugars may provoke inflammation. So may corn, especially if there is allergic cross-reactivity to corn products as found in high-fructose corn syrup (HFCS) sweetened soft drinks.

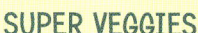

SUPER VEGGIES

Cruciferous vegetables (crucifers) such as arugula, bok choy, broccoli, Brussels sprouts, cabbage, cauliflower, collard greens, kale, kohlrabi, mizuna, mustard greens, radish greens, and turnip greens are considered anti-inflammatory superstars.

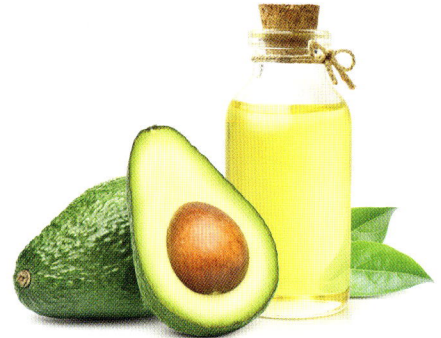

FATS AND OILS

The most favorable anti-inflammatory fats and oils are rich in monounsaturated fatty acids and/or omega-3-fatty acids.

Monounsaturated fatty acids found in avocados, nuts, and canola and olive oils, may be protective against cardiovascular disease and certain cancers and may improve insulin sensitivity. Nuts and nut "butters" such as almonds, hazelnuts, and walnuts and their oils are good sources of mono- and polyunsaturated fatty acids (including omega-3 fatty acids and antioxidant vitamin E) that may protect against harmful free radicals and reduce inflammation. Specifically, almonds, hazelnuts, and pecans provide excellent sources of vitamin E.

Omega-3 fatty acids found in cold-water fish, flaxseeds, omega-3 enriched eggs, walnuts, and

SORTING OUT SEEDS

Seeds and seed "butters" that include chia and freshly-ground flaxseeds are high in omega-3 fatty acids and lignans, phytochemicals with antioxidant properties. While hemp seeds tend to be higher in omega-6 fatty acids than other seeds, they contain gamma linoleic acid (GLA) that is considered anti-inflammatory.

whole-soy foods, may inhibit an enzymatic pathway that produces prostaglandins that activate pain, trigger inflammation, and defend the body against disease.

In contrast, omega 6-fatty acids, found in oils such as corn, safflower, soy, sunflower, and vegetable and their products may trigger the body to produce pro-inflammatory substances.

Use: Non-GMO canola and olive oil with anti-inflammatory omega-3 fatty acids. Canola and extra virgin olive oil are mostly comprised of oleic acid, a mono-unsaturated fatty acid that is associated with reduced blood pressure and LDL (bad) cholesterol and increased HDL (good) cholesterol. Olive oil is also a rich source of polyphenols with anti-inflammatory and antioxidant properties.

Limit: Corn, coconut, safflower, sesame, soy, and sunflower oils and hemp seeds with some pro-inflammatory omega-6 fatty acids should be limited.

Avoid: Butter, lard and margarine, the skin on poultry, and the fat that surrounds some meats contain saturated fatty acids that may raise total blood cholesterol and LDL (bad) cholesterol. These blood markers are of particular concern for people with arthritis who may also have greater risk of heart disease.

Trans fats may be found in very small amounts in beef and dairy products and some baked goods and fried foods. Most trans fats are formed when hydrogen is added to vegetable oils in the hydrogenation process and may trigger inflammation.

PROTEINS

Lean proteins may help to stabilize blood sugar and curtail inflammation. Focus on vegetable proteins, especially from legumes and soybeans and vitamin and mineral-rich nuts and seeds, along with fish with omega-3 fatty acids. Emphasize fresh protein-rich foods and minimize or eliminate processed proteins and fast foods.

Use: Incorporate lower-fat protein sources with their notable anti-inflammatory substances: fermented, probiotic dairy products (especially kefir and yogurt), legumes, and fish (especially sockeye

LOVING LEGUMES

Legumes such as Anasazi, adzuki, black, kidney and navy beans, black-eyed peas, chickpeas, and lentils are rich in folic acid, magnesium, potassium, and soluble fibers that help stabilize blood sugar levels. Legumes are also good-to-excellent sources of B-vitamins, calcium, iron, protein, zinc, and phytochemicals that help limit inflammation.

salmon and sardines). Soy foods—edamame, miso, tempeh, and tofu—contain fibers, polyunsaturated fatty acids, protein, vitamins, and minerals. Soy foods are low in saturated fats and contain phytosterols that may help lower LDL cholesterol.

Limit: Grass-fed, free-range, and organic lean meats (beef, lamb, and pork), and cage-free organic and skinless poultry tend to have higher levels of anti-inflammatory omega-3 fatty acids and lower levels of pro-inflammatory omega-6 fatty acids than protein foods produced other ways. Shellfish that include clams, lobster, oysters, mussels, and scallops tend to be higher in cholesterol and might generate or exacerbate gouty arthritis.

Avoid: Bacon, higher-fat cuts of beef such as corned beef, sausages, and spareribs; full-fat dairy products such as butter, cheese, cream, half-and-half, and ice cream; higher-fat foods with saturated and/or trans fatty acids, such as fried chicken or French fries; meats that are not free-range, grass-fed, or organic; processed meats (sandwich meats and sausages); and meat alternatives (veggie burgers and crumbles) may encourage inflammation as may peanuts in allergy-prone individuals.

FLUIDS

Although acute and chronic inflammation may be accompanied by swelling from the accumulation of body fluids, this does not mean that fluids should be restricted. On the contrary, water has many vital bodily functions. Hydration fights inflammation by flushing toxins out of the body, keeping the joints well-lubricated, and supporting weight loss.

Use: Natural mineral and spring water and water flavored with citrus or natural extracts. Water carries nutrients and oxygen to and through the blood and maintains water balance, internal body temperature, and moisture. It naturally suppresses the appetite, assists in metabolism of stored body fat, and transports by-products of fat metabolism for disposal.

At least 8 to 10 (8-ounce) glasses of natural or spring water (or naturally-flavored water) should be consumed daily depending upon individual needs, conditions and disease states, medications, and recommendations of health care providers.

THE DANGERS OF DEHYDRATION

Dehydration may lead to dizziness, dry hair, mouth and skin, headaches, increased thirst, decreased urine output and at its worst, confusion, low blood pressure, rapid heart rate, or even coma, seizure, or death. For some short term cures for dehydration, check out pages 107–109.

Limit: Alcohol, coffee and tea. There's not a clear scientific consensus, but alcohol may have both benefits and disadvantages. On the plus side, some alcoholic beverages (such as red wine with antioxidants) may help to improve insulin sensitivity, raise HDL (good) cholesterol, reduce blood clotting, and improve cardiovascular health. On the negative side, alcohol consumption may be counter-indicated and non-tolerated in certain ethnic populations. For example, some Eastern Asian people produce elevated amounts of acetaldehyde, a potentially toxic by-product of alcohol metabolism, with side effects that may include flushing, headache, nausea, and higher incidence of esophageal cancer. Also on the negative side are tannins in red wine with their astringency that may lead to headaches in some prone individuals.

Coffee contains phytochemicals that might reduce inflammation. Caffeine, a bitter-tasting alkaloid in coffee, is a central nervous system and cardiac stimulator. Moderate coffee consumption may be beneficial for cardiovascular health. However, coffee contains tannins like teas that may produce adverse gastrointestinal effects.

White, green, and oolong teas are rich in catechins, antioxidants that may help reduce inflammation. In particular, pure green (unfermented) tea leaves generally contain antioxidant-rich polyphenols, such as epigallocatchin gallate.

Avoid: Sugared beverages and diet sodas. Sugared beverages such as cocoa, fruit "-ades" such as lemonade, soft drinks, smoothies, sweetened alcoholic drinks, and sweetened coffee and tea mixes may promote inflammation. Diet sodas with artificial and natural sweeteners may still induce increased insulin response and may trigger weight gain, increased obesity risks (such as diabetes and heart disease), and other inflammatory conditions.

Other Inflammatory and Anti-Inflammatory Substances

Substances other than those found in major nutrients and water may be helpful in preventing and/or alleviating some inflammation symptoms. In addition to some coffees and teas, these include chocolate and various herbs and spices. Other substances, such as salt, may be sources of inflammation where indicated.

DARK CHOCOLATE

Dark chocolate with at least 70 percent cocoa contains antioxidants such as flavanols that may help to reduce inflammation and maintain healthy endothelial cells that line the arteries. Dark chocolate may also benefit cardiovascular function by improving arterial blood flow and reducing blood pressure, enhancing insulin sensitivity, and boosting healthy bacteria in the gastrointestinal tract.

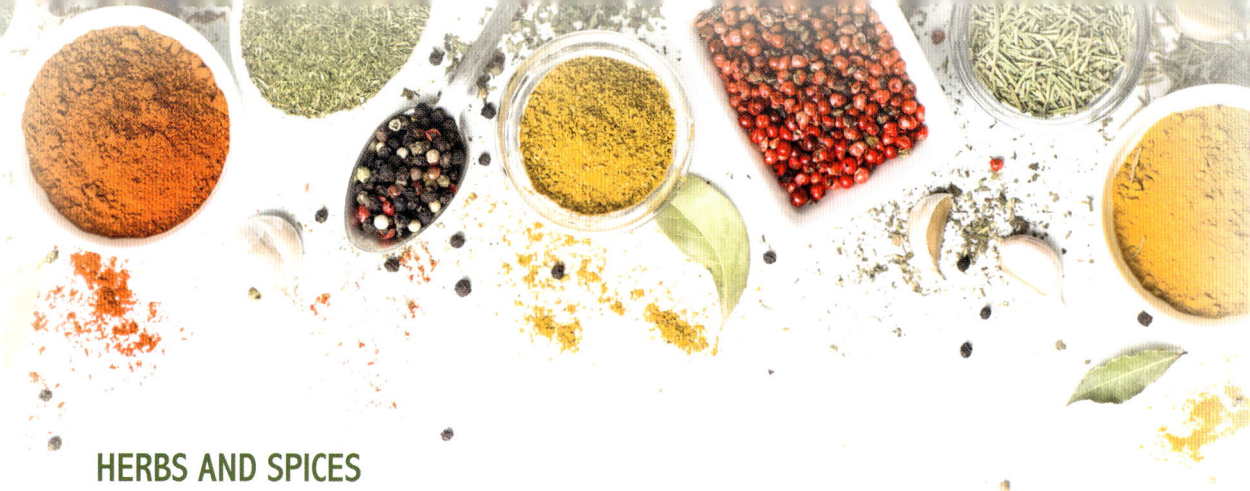

HERBS AND SPICES

Allspice contains analgesic, antibacterial, anti-inflammatory, and antioxidant substances. Allspice contains eugenol, quercetin, and tannins that help neutralize free radicals and counteract cellular mutations. Allspice might alleviate some arthritis, gout, hemorrhoids, and muscular aches and pains related to injuries and surgical recovery. Allspice may support dental health and maintain healthy digestion.

Black pepper contains piperine, an alkaloid found in the outer skin of pepper "berries" and jalapeño peppers. Piperine may boost the effectiveness of curcumin absorption (see turmeric). Black pepper is commonly used for gastrointestinal motility disorders.

Cayenne found in chili peppers contains capsaicinoids, alkaloids with pain-reduction and anti-inflammatory properties.

Cloves contain antibacterial, anti-inflammatory, and antioxidant benefits. Cloves may act as an anti-inflammatory for the mouth and throat, expectorant, and remedy for nausea and upset stomach. Cloves contain kaempferol and rhamnetin, flavonoids with similar properties to eugenol, an antiseptic and anti-inflammatory that may protect against cardiovascular disease by inhibiting abnormal blood platelet clotting.

Cinnamon contains cinnamaldehyde, a compound that may inhibit certain pro-inflammatory proteins and prevent blood platelet clotting. Cinnamon may help activate insulin receptors that assist blood sugar control. Cinnamon might block growth factors that are involved in abnormal cell growth and may be protective against certain cancers.

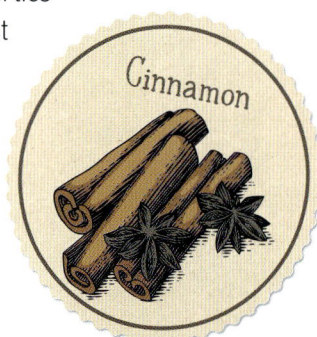

Food Pharmacy

Ginger contains antioxidant vitamin C, gingerol and shogoal, phenols that may help block inflammatory pathways. Ginger may act as an intestinal spasmolytic that relaxes and soothes the intestinal tract. Ginger might help reduce some osteoarthritis symptoms as a pain reliever and some side effects associated with chemotherapy.

Marjoram contains vitamins A, C, and K and may contain analgesic, anti-inflammatory, and antioxidant properties. Marjoram may support bone health and help reduce pain associated with arthritis, colds, fevers, headaches, muscular overexertion, spasms, and toothaches. Marjoram might also improve digestion by stimulating digestive enzymes.

Nutmeg contains pain-relieving properties from its volatile oils that include elemicin, eugenol, myristicin, and safrole. Nutmeg may help calm the digestive and nervous systems due to its B-vitamins, calcium, copper, iron, magnesium, manganese, and potassium content. Nutmeg might also aid blood pressure regulation and heart function.

Parsley contains rich sources of antioxidants and flavonoids. Parsley is an excellent source of vitamin C and a good source of vitamin A (notably from its beta-carotene content) and folic acid, an important B-vitamin for its anti-inflammatory properties for arthritis control and cardiovascular health. The flavonoids in parsley, particularly luteolin, may combat oxygen radicals to thwart cellular damage and increase the antioxidant capacity of the blood.

Rosemary contains anti-bacterial, anti-fungal, anti-inflammatory, antioxidant, and antiseptic properties.

Oregano contains betacaryophyllin that may help inhibit inflammation, resist bowel inflammation associated with Crohn's disease, and prevent bone degeneration associated with osteoarthritis.

Sage contains carnosic acid and carnosol, two anti-inflammatories that fight inflammation associated with certain neurological conditions, and camphor that may help destroy bacteria, fungi, and other compounds that may be effective antivirals.

Thyme contains carvacrol, a phenol that may suppress inflammatory enzymes, inhibit oxidative damage, and improve aches and muscles soreness. Thyme may also function as an antibacterial, antibiotic, antihistamine, and antiphylactic.

> Food colorings may trigger allergic reactions and other immune responses. Synthetic colorant molecules are small and the immune system may find them difficult to discern and defend. Colorants may also bind to food or proteins in the body and evade or disrupt the immune system.

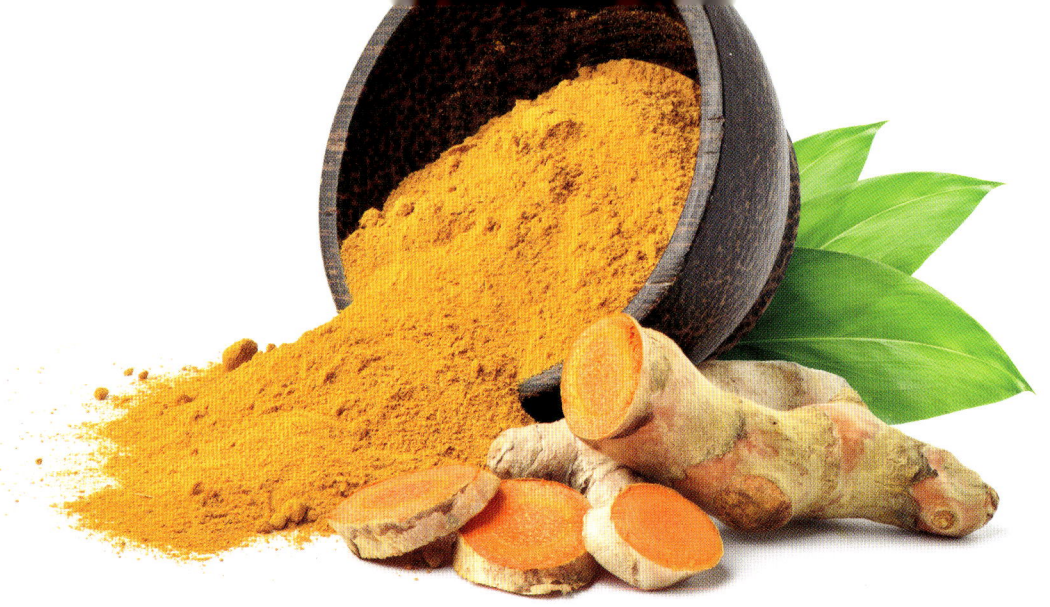

Turmeric, a member of the ginger family, contains the phenol curcuminoid. Curcumin, the most important curcuminoid, has antioxidant and anti-inflammatory effects. Turmeric may be effective in reducing inflammation associated with arthritis and diabetes and in some cancer prevention.

WHAT ABOUT SALT?

While sodium (a component of table salt) is an essential mineral in the human body for muscle contraction and relaxation, electrolyte balance, and nerve transmittance, too much sodium is counter-indicated for inflammation. When the kidneys cannot eliminate sodium effectively or speedily, sodium may accumulate in the blood stream, increase blood pressure, and stress the heart, kidneys, and liver. Excess sodium may also exacerbate certain inflammatory conditions, such as arthritis, that may cause blood vessels to expand and place pressure on surrounding joints. Corticosteroids used to treat rheumatoid arthritis may add to sodium retention, so excess salt may complicate their use.

SUPPLEMENTS AND MEDICATIONS

Ideally, dietary management should be able to alleviate and maybe dismiss some inflammatory symptoms. However, some people may have certain medical conditions that may require additional therapies. Supplements and medications should be individualized according to dietary and medical needs and monitored by health care practitioners.

Shopping and Preparing Meals

A well-stocked kitchen that supports an anti-inflammatory diet is essential for effective, healthy, and quick meals and snacks. Stock your pantry with whole and ancient grains, anti-inflammatory spices, and staples like nut butter. Clean your refrigerator frequently and stock it with fresh vegetables, fruits, and unsalted nuts and seeds.

Farm-raised, grass-fed, in-season, organic foods and beverages have gone mainstream at large and small markets and online. Ensure that their sources are accurate and reliable. Purchase staples that are devoid of sugars and other pro-inflammatory substances when they are on sale. Watch for weekly sales of anti-inflammatory protein foods and freeze in portion-controlled amounts. If you purchase extra fresh fruits, herbs, and/or vegetables, they may be "repurposed" into compotes, dressings, salads, sauces, soups, stews, and other preparations.

FOOD AND NUTRITION LABELS

Food and nutrition labels are meant to assist anti-inflammatory food and beverage selections, not to create alarm. In general, you should AVOID food with labels listing terms ending with "-ose" and other sugar-like substances.

If you are gluten-intolerant, be aware that the term "gluten-free" on food labels means that products still have less than 20 ppm of gluten. Watch out for barley, brewer's yeast, malt, oats, rye, triticale, and wheat even if they are labeled "gluten-free" and for the term "wheat-free" that may contain other undesirable and possibly disagreeable substances.

PLANNING MEALS

Every person needs to find the balance that works best for them, but in general, it is best to have three balanced meals daily with mini-snacks to help manage blood sugar and weight. Balancing meals around vitamin and mineral-rich vegetables and fruits, lean proteins, hearty carbohydrates, and healthy fats are a good starting point. Make vegetables a prominent feature of most meals. Fresh ingredients are usually best.

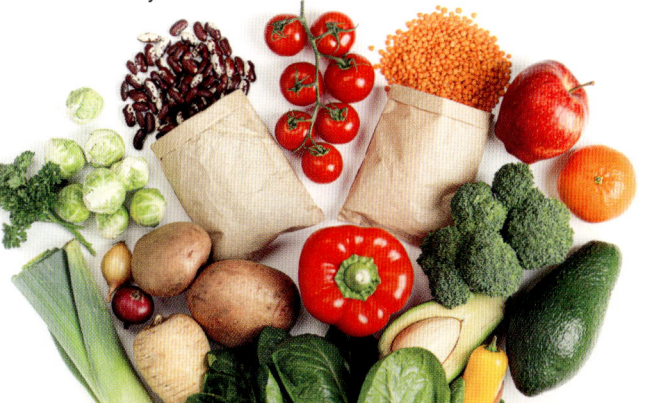

HOW YOU EAT

It's now just what you eat—it's how. It's important to eat and drink mindfully to help alleviate stressful eating. Slow down and enjoy dining experiences. Place silverware down between bites and sip. Don't gulp beverages. Chew and swallow food well and try to avoid "downing" food with liquids. Meals and snacks that are consumed on-the-run may not be best for proper digestion. Chronic stressful eating along with everyday pressures may overstress cortisol levels that may increase inflammation.

PUTTING IT ALL TOGETHER

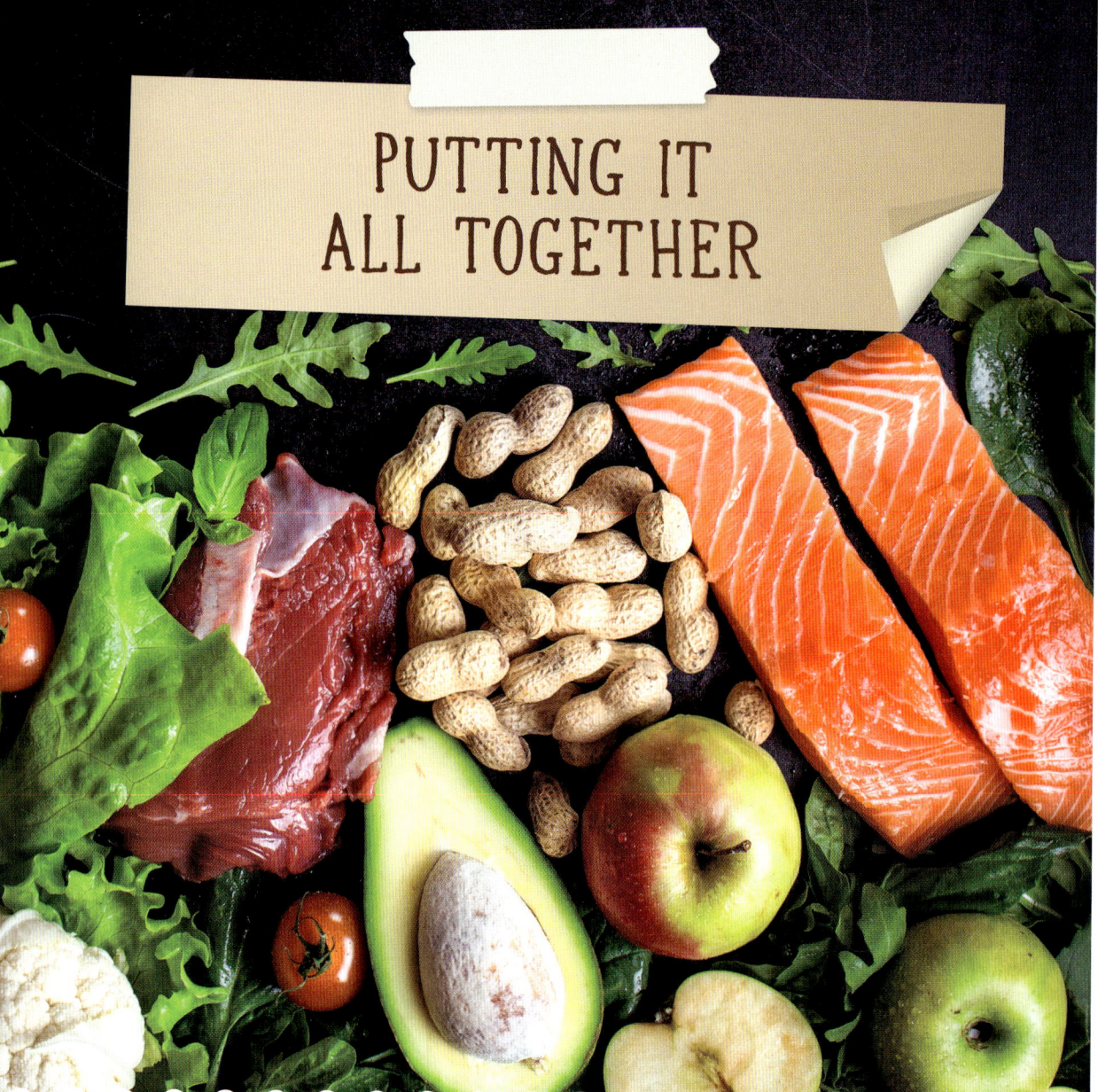

We've looked at specific vitamins and anti-inflammatory foods, but rather than focusing on a few foods or specific vitamins, the most important thing is to establish an overall pattern of healthy eating, one that will preserve the health of your heart, blood vessels, and brain. While there are no miracle foods, that doesn't mean that there aren't foods and nutrients that may be especially helpful. In this chapter, we'll look at a few specific diets that are associated with both heart health and brain health. First, let's look at some general guidelines that all these diets share.

The Threat of Atherosclerosis

Your blood vessels are essentially tubes made of living tissue that are lined on the inside with a layer of tissue called the endothelium. The blood vessel walls start out strong and flexible, with endothelium that is smooth and unblemished, allowing blood to flow through freely and easily as the heart's contractions pump it around the body. As the years go by, however, a condition called atherosclerosis, or hardening of the arteries, can occur. Hardening of the arteries is a very common condition that often begins to develop before we even reach our teens and slowly progresses over time.

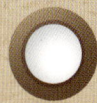

ATHEROSCLEROSIS AND AGE

Most often, atherosclerosis begins to seriously threaten the brain, the heart, or other organs when we reach our 50s and 60s.

Hardening of the arteries develops when damage to the endothelium leads to a buildup of cholesterol, fats, calcium, fibrin (which plays a role in blood clotting), and other substances on the inner walls of the arteries. These deposits, which are typically covered by a hard outer layer, are called plaques. As plaque builds up, it narrows the arteries, threatening the cells and organs that depend on those blood vessels to deliver life-giving blood. And when such narrowing occurs in the blood vessels that feed the brain, the brain's nerve cells can be jeopardized.

Variety, Balance, and Moderation

These are the watchwords of a healthy diet for your cardiovascular and brain health. Your brain, like the rest of your body, requires a plethora of nutrients—such as carbohydrates, protein, fat, vitamins, and minerals—to be healthy and to function well. Because no one food or group of foods can supply all of these nutrients, the best way to ensure that you give your brain everything it needs is to provide it with a variety of healthy foods.

Plant-based foods, in particular, offer the body all sorts of phytonutrients—substances that appear to have protective effects on the body's tissues and organs. Scientists have only just begun to identify and study the many phytonutrients thought to be supplied by plant foods. And while each of these substances appears to provide benefits on its own, experts believe that they are likely most effective when consumed together in the proportions found in actual foods. Since we don't know how phytonutrients work together, scientists recommend that you primarily get your nutrients from food, not from supplements.

Your body not only needs a wide assortment of nutrients, it needs them in balance. Getting too little or too much of certain nutrients can throw others out of whack and actually hinder the way the body functions. Once again, the best way to include the proper balance your brain and body need is to consume nutrients in their natural containers—whole foods in as close to their natural state as possible.

And finally, going hand in hand with balance is moderation. Too much of anything is no good, as they say, and it's true when you're eating for heart and brain health. Even water, that life-giving fluid, can be dangerous if consumed in extremes. And while you may decide to swear off forever certain favorite foods because of their potential negative effects on your body, you'll be more likely to stay with your healthy dietary changes if you allow yourself the occasional treat. After all, nothing makes us want something more than being told that we can never have it again. So stay away from words like "never," allow yourself the rare treat, and remember that moderation is the key to enjoyable success.

> ### A QUICK CAUTION
>
> Before making any significant changes in your diet or activity level, it's always best to discuss your plans with your doctor and get the OK first. And if you're under the care of more than one physician—because of a chronic condition such as heart disease, high blood pressure, or diabetes, for example—be sure to check with each doctor.

Beets

WHOLE GRAINS, BEANS, FRESH FRUITS, AND VEGGIES

Whole grains and legumes, along with fruits and vegetables, tend to be rich in nutrients, high in complex carbohydrates and fiber, and low in fat and cholesterol, so they deliver a lot of nutritional bang for your calorie buck. A diet in which these foods are center stage has been associated with a lower risk of stroke, heart and blood vessel disease, high blood cholesterol and triglycerides, high blood pressure, and diabetes.

Their carbohydrate content provides a ready source of energy for the body. And the fiber content of these plant foods is a boon to weight control. Fiber passes through the body without being broken down, so it doesn't supply your body with any calories. That means you can eat larger and more filling portions of these foods without maxing out your calorie budget. Fiber also acts as nature's broom, binding with and removing excess blood cholesterol from the body and keeping food and waste moving smoothly through the digestive tract.

Their generally low fat content comes from unsaturated fats, which are better for your brain.

They provide a variety of amino acids, from which protein is made. Protein plays many roles in the brain (and throughout the body), including the relay of messages between neurons. And finally, these foods are packed with essential vitamins and minerals and countless phytonutrients that benefit the brain.

EMPHASIZING VARIETY

Eating a wide variety of foods is a way to ensure that your brain and body get plenty of the essential nutrients and protective phytonutrients that can help keep them functioning well as the years go by. That advice is just as important when it comes to fruits and vegetables.

AN EASY METHOD

To help ensure that you're getting enough of these valuable foods, you don't need to count calories. One simple method is to just make sure that at meals, you're filling up at least half, and up to two-thirds, of your plate with them. Treat meat, fats, and dairy as add-ons and accent foods, instead of always putting them front and center.

Many kinds of produce provide vitamin C, beta-carotene (a form of vitamin A), flavonoids, and/or other phytonutrients that have anti-inflammatory and antioxidant powers. Inflammation is thought to be a major contributor to hardening of the arteries, which can compromise the blood flow to the brain. Inflammation likely also plays some role in the development of Alzheimer's disease. Anti-inflammatory compounds in fruits and vegetables fight against such inflammation.

Antioxidant compounds in foods help to defend the body's cells, including those in the brain and blood-vessel lining, from damage caused by oxidation (the same process that causes metal to rust). Oxidation occurs naturally in the body, as cells use oxygen for various functions, but it also results from exposure to toxins and other insults, such as cigarette smoke and certain illegal drugs and air pollutants. The body uses antioxidants to protect its cells from such damage, but sometimes the oxidative stress overwhelms the body's defensive resources, causing cell damage that can eventually lead to stroke, heart disease, cancer, or other medical problems. Consuming a diet rich in antioxidants helps to strengthen the body's defenses and so may prevent or lessen physical deterioration in the brain due to aging.

In general, the deeper or darker the color of the produce, the greater its phytonutrient content. Fruits that fall into this category include berries, cherries, red grapes, raisins, plums and prunes, and oranges and nectarines. Examples of dark- or deep-colored vegetables include broccoli, brussels sprouts, spinach, kale, beets, corn, onions, and peppers.

Berries may be especially beneficial as a fruit, since research indicates that eating lots of blueberries and strawberries appears to slow cognitive decline in older folks, delaying it by as much as 2.5 years. Both fruits are loaded with phytonutrients called flavonoids that have anti-inflammatory and antioxidant powers. Getting more total flavonoids was also associated with an actual reduction in the degeneration of cognitive function that typically occurs as we age.

COUNT TO 30

One study suggested that people who ate 30 different plant-based foods a week had more gut microbes, one key to overall health, than those who ate ten or fewer. This number included grains and seeds; in a multi-grain bread, you would count each different grain type towards your number.

WHAT NOT TO EAT

Candy, pastries, donuts, cakes, ice cream, and soda and other sugary beverages provide lots of calories in the form of simple sugars, but these foods typically provide little else of nutritional value. So including them frequently in the diet is essentially a waste of calories.

What's more, many of these sweet treats also include saturated and trans fats, two types of fat that can contribute to hardening of the arteries. You're far better off spending your daily calorie budget on foods that actually supply those nutrients. Use fresh, ripe fruit to satisfy your sweet tooth, and keep the sugary foods and beverages filled with empty calories for the occasional treat.

EATING FATS WISELY

Despite its bad reputation, fat is a fundamental element of the body as a whole. It plays a variety of useful roles and is an essential part of a healthy diet. Problems arise when we take in far more fat than we need and when we choose foods that are packed with potentially harmful types of fats.

Unlike the carbohydrates and protein we consume, which supply four calories per gram, dietary fat supplies nine calories per gram. It's a concentrated form of stored energy, which makes it extremely valuable during times of food shortage or famine. But these days, most of us in the United States suffer because we take in too many calories, not too few. A high intake of fat has been linked to overweight and obesity, which can increase the risk of conditions such as high blood pressure and diabetes.

Research has also linked a high-fat diet—specifically one that is high in saturated and trans fats—to high levels of bad (LDL) cholesterol, low levels of good (HDL) cholesterol, and an increased risk of stroke and heart disease.

Saturated fats and trans fats both tend to be solid at room temperature. Saturated fats occur naturally in animal products, such as red meat, poultry, and full-fat dairy products. Trans fats are primarily found in many commercially prepared cookies, pastries, pie crusts, crackers, pizza dough, baked goods, fried foods, and stick margarines (although a backlash against these fats by consumer groups has prompted some food companies to remove trans fats from their products).

While trans fats occur naturally in minimal amounts in some foods, most trans fats in the American diet are created by the food industry from oils that are put through a process called partial hydrogenation; partially hydrogenating oils increases their shelf life and makes them easier to cook with.

A diet that is healthy for cells throughout the body should instead include a moderate amount (between 20 and 30 percent or so of total calories) of monounsaturated and polyunsaturated fats, especially polyunsaturated fats that are high in a type of fatty acid called omega-3. Research indicates that a diet in which olive oil—which is rich in monounsaturated fats—contributes the vast majority of fat may help prevent age-related memory loss in healthy older people. The more of this type of fat the subjects consumed, the greater the protection. Monounsaturated fat also appears to have a protective effect on the heart and blood vessels.

Similarly, polyunsaturated fats, particularly those that are high in omega-3 fatty acids, appear to benefit the health of the brain and body in a variety of ways. Research suggests that these fatty acids, found most abundantly in cold-water fish, may help lower the risk of high blood pressure, stroke, and heart disease.

Polyunsaturated fats, like their monounsaturated cousins, tend to be liquid at room temperature. Omega-3 fatty acids are found in certain plant foods, including walnuts, sunflower seeds and sunflower oil, soybeans and soybean oil, canola oil, and ground flaxseed, although the body can't use them as well as the omega-3s that come from fish.

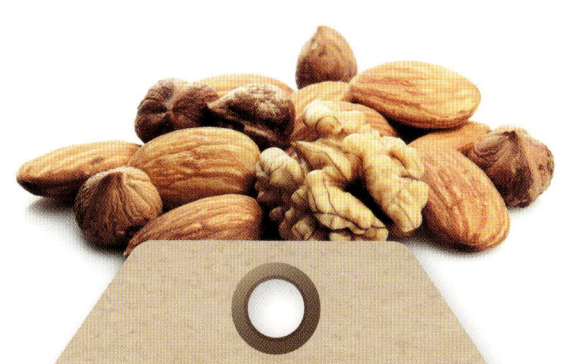

GO NUTS

A small handful of unsalted nuts, including almonds, hazelnuts, pecans, pine nuts, peanuts (which are actually legumes, not true nuts), and/or walnuts makes a great brain-smart snack. They're a good source of filling protein and a great source of vitamin E, an antioxidant that can help shield your brain cells from damage. Plus, most of their fat is the beneficial monounsaturated variety.

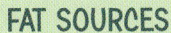

FAT SOURCES

Foods that contain mostly monounsaturated fats include olives and olive oil, canola and sunflower oils, nuts, and avocado.

INCREMENTAL CHANGES

The following tips can help you begin to lower your total fat intake and replace unhealthy saturated and trans fats with beneficial unsaturated fats:

- Trim the visible marbling from meats, and choose leaner cuts, such as round and loin cuts, over well-marbled cuts such as rib and shoulder cuts. Keep in mind that when it comes to the grade of beef, veal, and lamb, "prime" cuts have the most fat, "choice" have less, and "good" the least.

- Limit fatty and salty luncheon meats and other high-fat processed meats, including hot dogs, bacon, and sausage; more than half their calories come from fat, and most of that is saturated.

- Trim the skin and visible fat from poultry, and limit goose and duck, which are very high in saturated fat.

- Choose fish (especially cold-water types); white-meat poultry without the skin; and beans, nuts, and other legumes more often than red meat and pork as your protein source in a meal. And try using meat as a topping or accent to pasta and rice dishes instead of making it the main entrée.

- Instead of frying meat and poultry, try baking, broiling, or roasting. When basting, use wine, lemon juice, or tomato juice instead of the fatty drippings from the meat or poultry itself.

- Purchase tuna or other fish packed in water rather than oil. If water-packed isn't available, rinse the fish before eating.

- Opt for fat-free and low-fat versions of dairy products, and try substituting plain nonfat yogurt for sour cream as a topping.

- Choose low-fat versions of foods when available, but before you put a product in your cart, compare the calories per serving of the low-fat and regular versions to be sure the low-fat version is actually lower in calories as well. (Some food manufacturers make up for the loss of flavor from fat by adding more sugar or salt.)

- Check your sauces and condiments; when you can, avoid eating whole grains, vegetables, fish, and lean meats with cream, butter, or cheese sauce.

FANTASTIC FISH

Cold-water fish rich in omega-3 fatty acids include herring, mackerel, salmon, sardines, trout, and tuna. Experts are so impressed with the protective effects of omega-3 fatty acids that many recommend that we choose cold-water fish as our protein source in two or three meals a week.

The Mediterranean Diet

What is the Mediterranean diet? It is a mostly commonsense approach to eating modeled on the eating habits of countries that border the Mediterranean Sea. These include European countries: Spain, France, Italy, and Greece; Middle Eastern countries: Turkey, Syria, and Lebanon; and African countries: Egypt, Libya, Tunisia, Algeria, and Morocco.

This diverse list of countries may not seem to have much in common at first, but as you examine the native cuisines of the people, a pattern emerges: an emphasis on fresh vegetables, fruit, whole grains, fish and seafood, healthy unsaturated fats, and smaller amounts of meat, dairy, and refined grains. Research that goes back as far as the 1950s indicates that people in these countries were exceptionally healthier and had lower risk to many lifestyle diseases, like heart attacks, strokes, and type 2 diabetes, based on their eating patterns and cooking styles. Both the DASH and MIND diets explored later in this chapter have a lot in common with the Mediterranean diet.

There is a lifestyle component as well, a mindful approach to meals. Minimize distractions (phones, television, etc.), focusing instead on eating slowly and enjoying every bite.

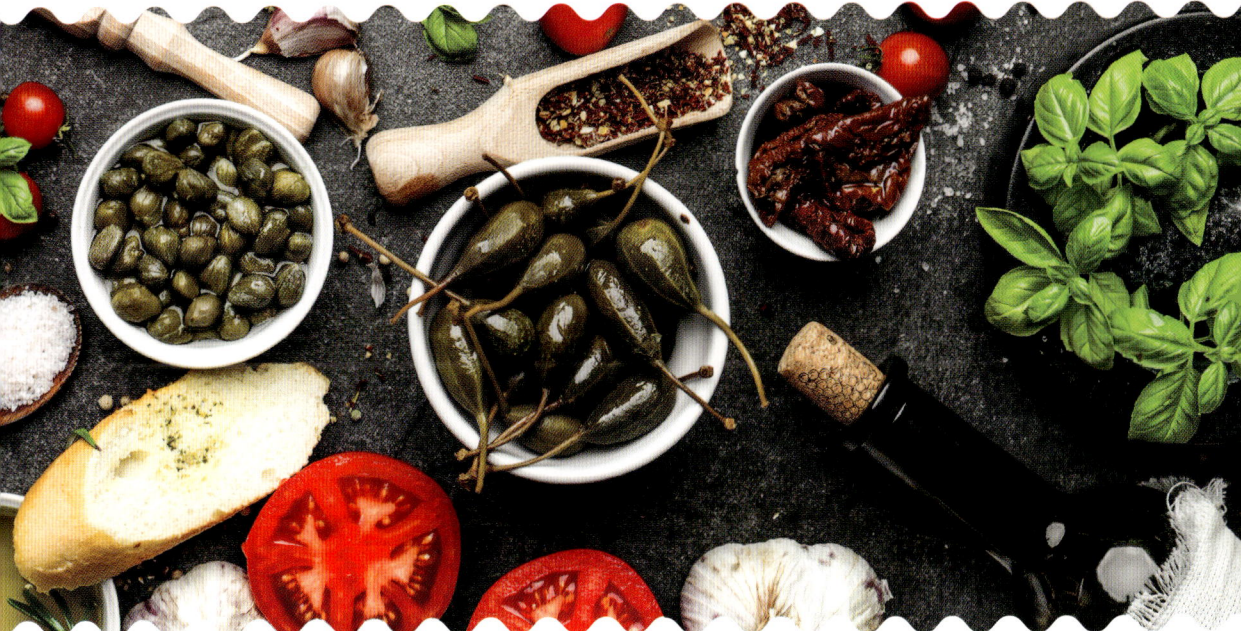

HOW TO EAT MEDITERRANEAN

The Mediterranean diet is primarily plant based, so plan on basing your meals on vegetables, fruit, grains, and legumes with a bit of dairy thrown in for seasoning. Add fish, seafood, or chicken a few times a week, and reserve red meat for occasional treats.

If reducing the amount of meat in your diet seems too difficult, start small and try one or two nights a week without it. As you can see from the Mediterranean food pyramid, there are plenty of delicious options. The basic guidelines are as follows:

What to Eat: A large variety of plant-based foods, including fruits (as desserts), vegetables, potatoes, whole grains, beans, nuts, legumes, and seeds

Mostly: Vegetables, fruits, nuts, seeds, legumes, potatoes, whole grains, breads, herbs, spices, fish, seafood, extra virgin olive oil

Moderately: Poultry (no more than twice/week) and fish, eggs (no more than 7/week, including those used in cooking), cheese, yogurt

Rarely: Red meat (no more than twice/month)

Avoid: Added sugars and sweets like candies, cookies, pastries, sweetened beverages; processed meats like hot dogs, sausages; refined grains and pasta; trans fats found in margarine and processed foods

Activity: Include daily physical activity and positive lifestyle choices

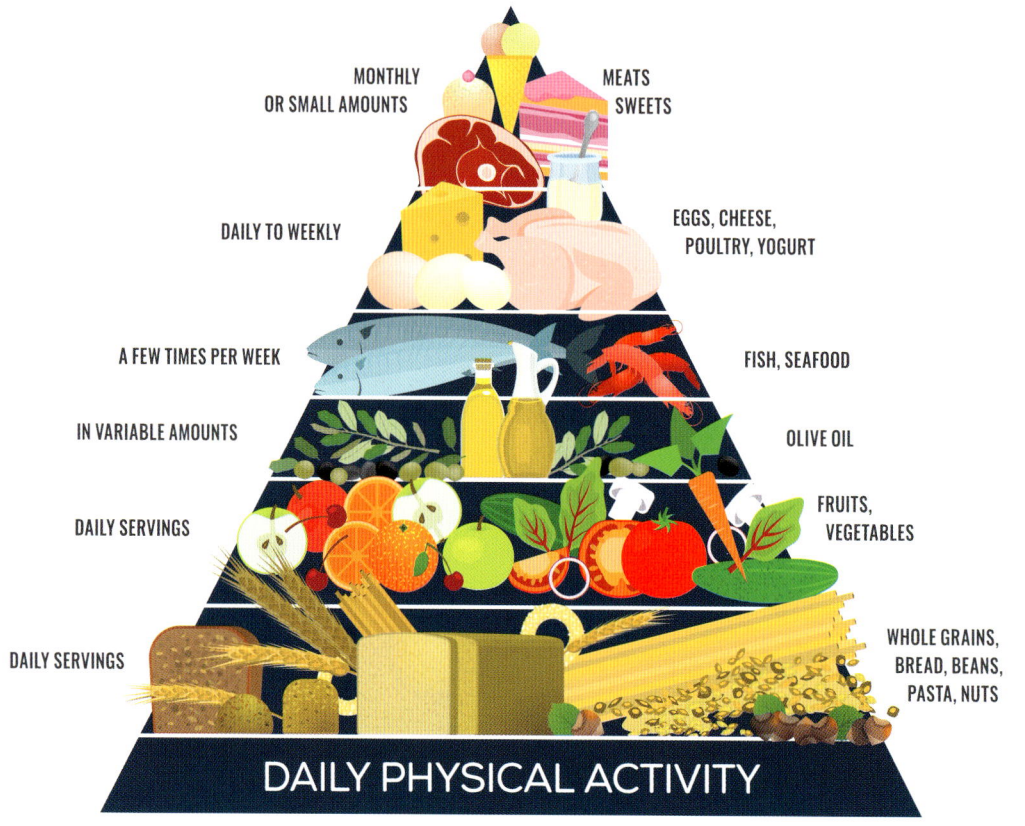

Food Pharmacy

GETTING STARTED AND STAYING ON TRACK

Get organized. Clean out your pantry and get rid of unhealthy snacks like chips, cookies, and candy and replace them with better choices like roasted nuts, olives, and fresh fruit like grapes, apples, and oranges. Plan your meals in advance, and try to pick things that have similar ingredients. It's easier to buy larger quantities of fewer items than it is to buy small quantities of more items. Also, it will help you stay focused and give you less to think about if you know that you're using, say, tomatoes, cucumbers, and onions for several meals rather than different ingredients every night.

Spend some time each week cleaning out your refrigerator. Check the status of your eggs, Greek yogurt, and cucumbers and keep a running list of what's running low. Discard any leftovers that are long past their prime, and plan a night to serve recent leftovers as a mezze spread. Mezze is a style of dining where small plates make up a meal, similar to tapas. Give it a try at the end of the week when you've got little bits of leftovers to use up—just buy or make some fresh pita, whip up a fresh salad and set out cold salads, grain dishes, and meats leftover from the week. Another fun idea is to serve dips, like hummus (chickpea spread), tzatziki (yogurt-based dip), or baba ghanoush (eggplant and sesame) with vegetables.

Keep rice, lentils, pasta, nuts, and cheese on hand. Not only will you need them to make many Mediterranean recipes, but they're great to have on hand for simple last-minute meals. Marinated feta, for example, is great to have on hand for snacking or adding to salads or pasta dishes.

Keep two kinds of olive oil on hand. Select a decent olive oil for sautéeing and cooking and a high-quality extra virgin olive oil for making dressings and sauces and using in other places where you'll really taste the flavor.

Try to make every meal an occasion. Eating should be an enjoyable experience that is a real part of your day, not just a task to be endured. Turn off distractions like televisions, phones, and tablets, and turn on music instead. Allow enough time that everyone can eat at their own pace without feeling rushed. If you need to train yourself to eat slower, put down your fork after every bite, and chew and swallow before picking it up again.

HEALTHY HYDRATION

While you're making good food decisions, make good beverage choices as well. Instead of sugary sodas and coffee drinks, try tea and coffee either black or with a splash of cream and a drizzle of honey (yes, even in coffee—it's good!). Instead of soda, try plain sparkling water mixed with a squeeze of fresh lime, lemon, or grapefruit juice. Or infuse regular water with cucumber, mint, and/or lemon; keep a pitcher in your refrigerator or stick a mint sprig and a lemon wedge in your water bottle for flavored water throughout the day.

Add in healthy foods. Add vegetables to pastas, stir fries, and soups. Add beans or chickpeas to salads, quesadillas, and tacos. Add pine nuts or slivered almonds to green beans or other vegetables or rice.

Overall, there is no one defined Mediterranean eating style. It's important to choose a plan that is rich in plant foods and lower in animal products and emphasize fish and seafood.

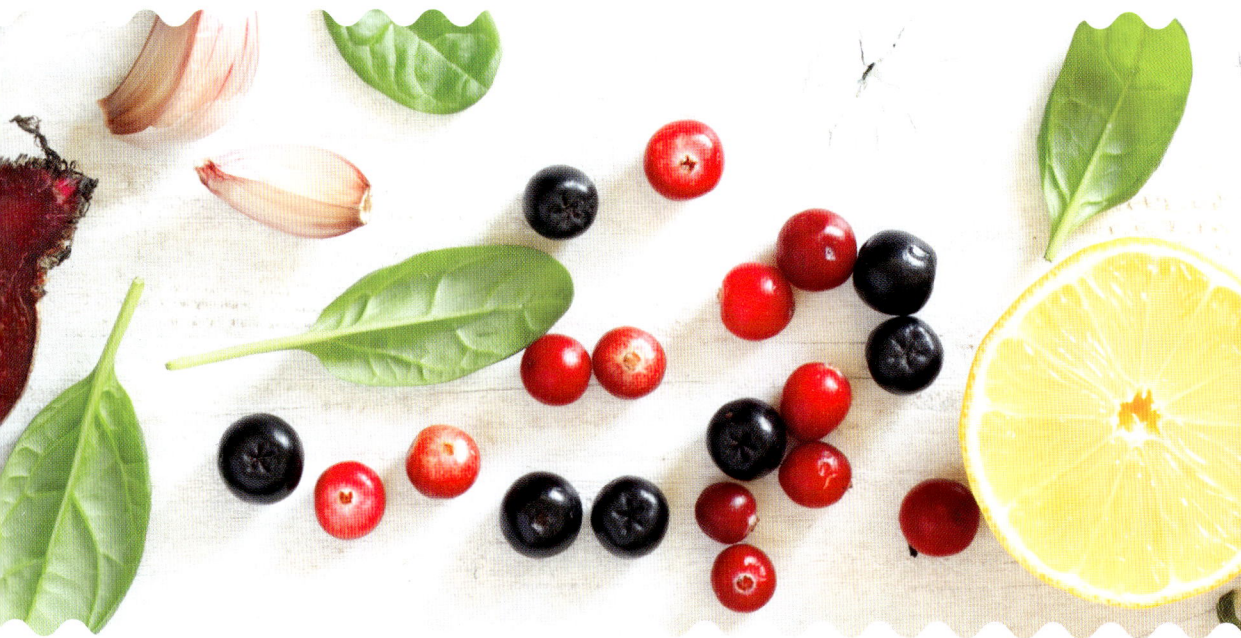

The DASH Diet

DASH stands for Dietary Approaches to Stop Hypertension. Although it sounds like the DASH diet can be done in a "dash", it's really the diet recommendations and the combination of foods and beverages of the DASH diet that lead to its success.

DASH DEVELOPMENT

The DASH diet was originally developed by the National Heart, Lung and Blood Institute (NHLBI) during a study to discover ways to reduce blood pressure without medication. The original diet was based on the best practices of vegetarian diets, since vegetables were known to lower blood pressure. But most Americans were meat eaters at the time, so the diet combined the best of both dietary approaches—vegetables plus lean meats and protein.

Not only did the DASH diet lower blood pressure, but it lowered cholesterol that was associated with heart disease, heart failure, kidney disease and kidney stones, some types of cancer, stroke, type 2 diabetes, and other conditions and diseases. And, the DASH diet led to weight loss since it was packed with bulky, filling and nutrient-rich fruits and vegetables, along with lean proteins for satisfaction and great taste.

Today, the DASH diet is promoted by US Dietary Guidelines for Americans. The US Dietary Guidelines are a tool for professionals to help Americans make healthy food and beverages choices to help prevent chronic diseases. The DASH diet has been highly ranked for years as one of the best diets. It is supported by research from numerous clinical trials, endorsed by the US government, and praised by doctors and nutritionists for its healthy recommendations and benefits.

BENEFITS

- The DASH diet is easy to follow, effective for weight loss, flexible, nutritious, and well-rounded. Plus, it is designed for present and future diet and weight loss success.

- The DASH diet focuses on healthy foods and beverages that lower blood pressure without medication. These include fish and seafood, fruits, legumes, lean meats and poultry, low-fat dairy products, and vegetables.

- The DASH diet recipes typically have fewer ingredients and contain common ingredients that are easy to find and don't require special cooking skills or equipment.

- The DASH diet helps reduce some conditions and diseases, such as diabetes, heart disease, hypertension, osteoporosis, some types of cancer, and stroke.

Hypertension may decrease in as little as 2 weeks on the DASH diet, depending upon individual differences.

WHAT IS THE BASIS OF THE DASH DIET?

It does not focus on strict portion sizes; the elimination of certain foods or beverages; or special foods, beverages, or supplements. Rather, it emphasizes eating the healthiest foods and beverages.

- The DASH diet features plenty of fruits, low-fat dairy products, and vegetables, along with fish and seafood, lean meats, nuts and seeds, poultry, and whole grains.

- Many of these foods and beverages tend to be lower in sodium and richer in calcium, magnesium, and potassium, to help lower blood pressure by promoting the relaxation of blood vessels and permitting blood to flow freely.

- Since the DASH diet is so balanced, it can lead to sustained weight loss.

- The DASH diet encourages the consumption of fruits and vegetables rich in dietary fiber that are filling and contribute to healthy digestion, and plant nutrients that are loaded with disease-fighting vitamins and minerals.

- The DASH diet focuses on moderate portion sizes so that calories are controlled. Think ½ + ¼ + ¼.
- Half of your plate should include fruits and vegetables (such as green leafy salad or cooked broccoli).
- One-quarter should come from higher-fiber whole grains (such as cooked brown rice or quinoa).
- One-quarter should come from lean proteins (such as grilled fish or skinless chicken breast).

The DASH diet also emphasizes the importance of regular physical activity into daily routines. This amounts to at least thirty minutes of walking 5 days a week, muscle-strengthening activities 2 or more days each week, and regular daily stretching to keep muscles limber.

THE DASH DIET GUIDELINES

The DASH diet guidelines closely duplicate the US Dietary Guidelines for Americans. This is why the DASH diet is considered so healthy and effective for weight loss and weight management.

- Choose low-fat and nonfat dairy products.
- Consume more fruits and vegetables.
- Substitute whole grains for refined grains.
- Limit added sugars.
- Limit saturated fats.
- Select lean protein sources.
- Use less salt and sodium. Limit sodium to 2,300 milligrams daily or less.
- Individuals with hypertension should aim for about 1,500 milligrams of sodium daily.

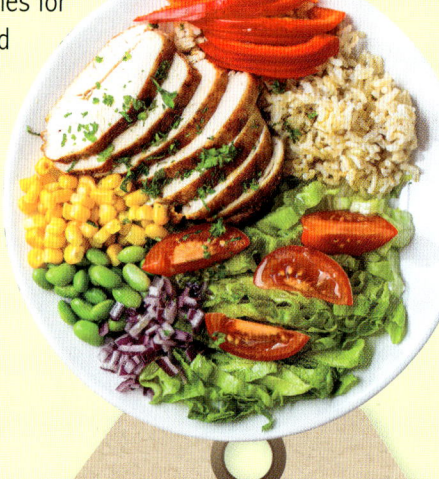

WHAT ABOUT ALCOHOL?
Alcohol, if consumed, should be used in moderation—up to one drink daily for women and up to two drinks daily for men, and only by adults of legal drinking age.

The US Dietary Guidelines for Americans suggest a healthy eating pattern that focuses on foods and beverages that are low in added sugars, saturated and trans fats, and sodium. Specifically, get less than 10% of total calories daily from added sugars; less than 10% of total calories daily from saturated fats; and less than 2,300 milligrams (mg) daily of sodium.

WHAT SHOULD I EAT ON THE DASH DIET?

The DASH diet recommends foods and beverages that focus on a number of daily servings from each of the major food groups.

Food or Beverage	Number of Servings	Serving Sizes
Fat-free or low-fat dairy products	2–3 servings daily	1 cup
Fats and oils	2–3 servings daily	1 teaspoon
Fruits	4–5 servings daily	½ cup or 1 medium fruit
Lean meat, poultry, fish	6 servings or fewer daily	1 ounce
Nuts, seeds, legumes	4–5 servings weekly	⅓ cup nuts or 2 tablespoons seeds or ½ cup cooked legumes
Vegetables	4–5 servings daily	½ cup cooked or 1 cup fresh
Grains	6–8 servings daily	1 slice bread or 1 ounce dry cereal or ½ cup cooked cereal, pasta or rice
Sweets	5 servings or fewer weekly	1 tablespoon jam, jelly, or sugar or ½ cup sorbet or 1 cup lemonade

SODIUM SWAP

Instead of Higher Sodium Foods...	Choose Lower Sodium Substitutes...
½ cup canned kidney beans (435mg)	½ cup cooked dried or frozen navy beans without salt (2mg)
1 cup ready-to-eat breakfast cereal (0-300mg)	½ cup unsalted cooked breakfast cereal (0-5mg)
½ cup canned corn (280mg)	½ cup cooked fresh corn kernels (4mg)
½ cup stewed tomatoes (282mg)	½ cup fresh chopped tomatoes (8mg)
1 cup low-fat chocolate milk (153mg)	1 cup skim milk (127mg)
1 ounce pasteurized processed cheese (409mg)	1 ounce part-skim mozzarella cheese (150mg)
2 tbsp. salted dry-roasted peanuts (230mg)	2 tbsp. unsalted dry roasted peanuts (2mg)
3 ounces cured ham (1,128mg)	3 ounces roast pork (54mg)
1 ounce salted potato chips (168mg)	1 ounce unsalted potato chips (2mg)
1 tbsp. blue cheese-type salad dressing (167mg)	1 tbsp. low-sodium blue cheese-type salad dressing (5mg)

Putting It All Together

USING THE NUTRITIONAL FACTS LABEL

The Nutrition Facts Label is a label that is required by the US Food and Drug Administration (FDA) on most packaged foods and beverages. It provides detailed information about the nutrient content of foods and beverages and helps consumers make more informed choices for disease prevention, health, and weight.

By using the Nutrition Facts Label consumers are able to see the number of calories per package and per serving with realistic serving sizes, added sugars, and other nutrients. The reason why the Nutrition Facts Label is an important tool for the DASH Diet is that it helps consumers compare and contrast foods and beverages to obtain the best nutrients for the least calories.

Two Nutrition Facts Labels are shown below. The first label (A) is for flour tortillas and the second label (B) for corn tortillas. A comparison of nutrients follow.

A

Nutrition Facts
10 servings per container
Serving size 1 tortilla (36g)

Amount Per Serving
Calories 110

	% Daily Value*
Total Fat 2.5g	3%
Saturated Fat 1g	5%
Trans Fat 0g	
Cholesterol 0mg	0%
Sodium 310mg	13%
Total Carbohydrate 18g	7%
Dietary Fiber 1g	4%
Total Sugars 0g	
Includes 0g Added Sugars	0%
Protein 3g	6%

Not a significant source of vitamin D, calcium, iron, and potassium

*The % Daily Value (DV) tells you how much a nutrient in a serving of food contributes to a daily diet. 2,000 calories a day is used for general nutrition advice.

B

Nutrition Facts
10 servings per container
Serving size 1 tortilla (30g)

Amount Per Serving
Calories 70

	% Daily Value*
Total Fat 1g	1%
Saturated Fat 0g	0%
Trans Fat 0g	
Cholesterol 0mg	0%
Sodium 5mg	0%
Total Carbohydrate 13g	5%
Dietary Fiber 2g	7%
Total Sugars 1g	
Includes 0g Added Sugars	0%
Protein 1g	2%

Not a significant source of vitamin D, calcium, iron, and potassium

*The % Daily Value (DV) tells you how much a nutrient in a serving of food contributes to a daily diet. 2,000 calories a day is used for general nutrition advice.

By comparing these two labels, it is easy to see by the highlighted values that the corn tortilla is lower in calories, total and saturated fat, sodium and carbohydrates, and higher in dietary fiber than the flour tortilla, therefore being a better choice.

LIVING A HEALTHY LIFESTYLE

While the DASH diet takes more than "a dash" of effort, just follow these recommendations for S.P.E.E.D.Y success!

- **S**hop Smartly—Compare nutrition labels.
- **P**rep Carefully—Don't add unnecessary fats, salt, or sugar.
- **E**at Wisely—Follow the DASH diet recommendations.
- **E**xercise Deliberately—Be intentionally active.
- **D**ecide Sensibly—Select foods to enjoy, limit others.
- **Y**ield Gently—Permit diet fallbacks, then get back on track for healthy living.

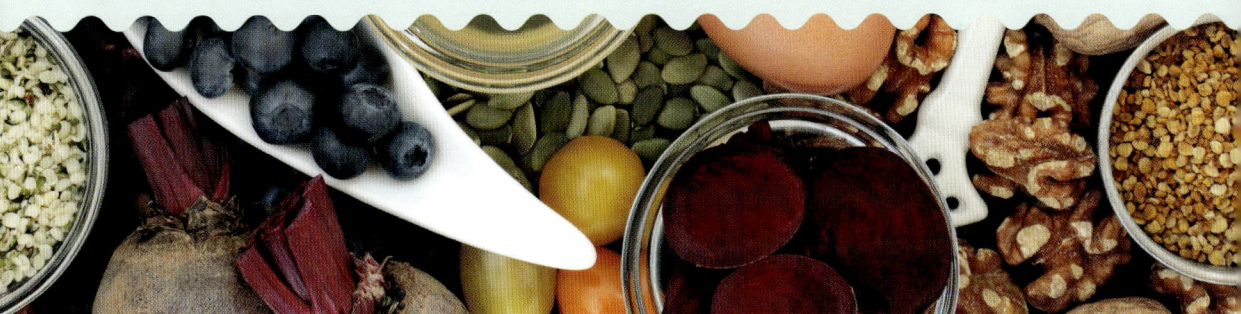

The MIND Diet

The MIND diet combines aspects of the Mediterranean and DASH diets, and specifically focuses on brain health. In fact, its full name is the Mediterranean-DASH Intervention for Neurodegenerative Delay (MIND) diet. Early research suggests that the MIND diet may reduce the risk of Alzheimer's disease and slow the decline in brain function that can happen with age.

The MIND diet encourages many of the plant-based foods recommended in the Mediterranean and DASH diets, as well as fish and poultry, while limiting saturated fats and added sugars. The MIND diet specifies the type and amount of fruits and vegetables to be consumed.

> The great news about the MIND diet is that you don't have to follow it perfectly to benefit. Adults in the study who followed the diet rigorously lowered their Alzheimer's risk by as much as 53 percent, while those who only followed it moderately well still cut their risk by about 35 percent.

Putting It All Together

FOODS TO EAT

Food or Beverage	Number of Servings
Green leafy vegetables	6 or more servings per week
Other vegetables	1 or more servings per day
Berries	2 or more servings per week
Whole grains	3 or more servings per day
Nuts	5 or more servings per week
Beans	4 or more servings per week
Poultry	2 or more servings per week
Fish	1 or more servings per week
Olive oil	use as cooking oil
Wine	no more than 1 glass per day

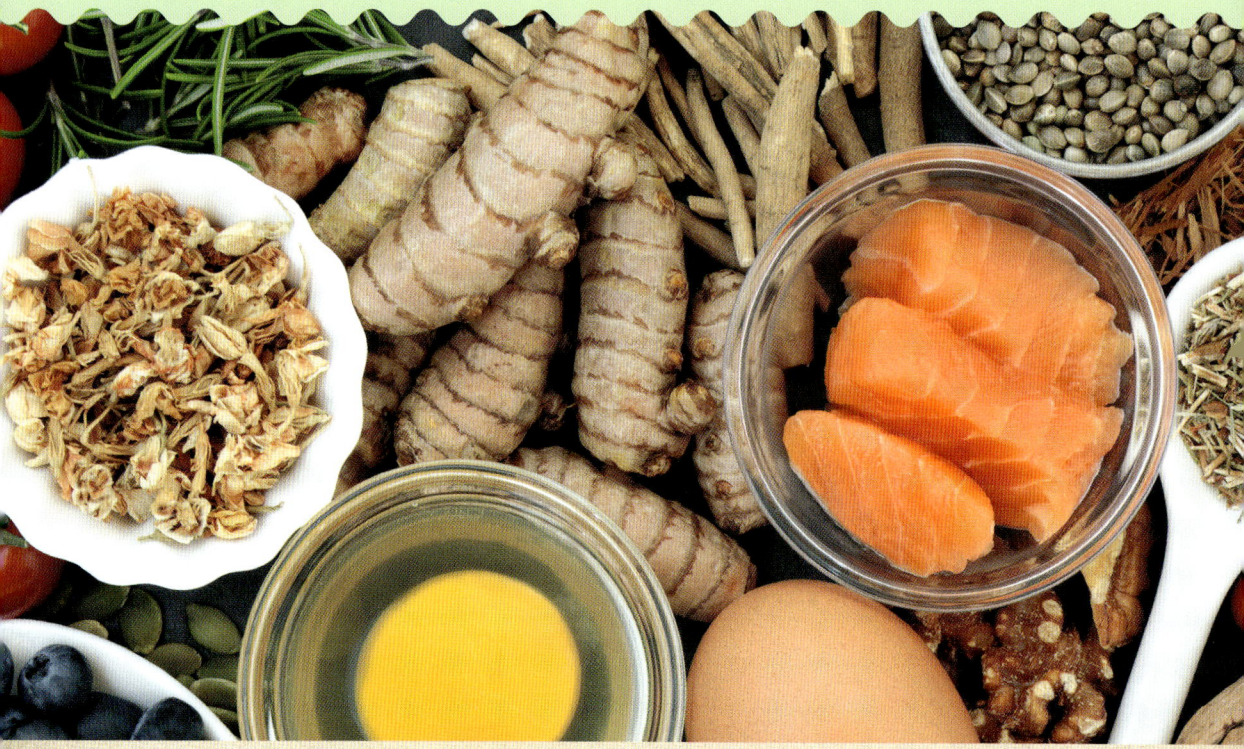

FOODS TO AVOID

Butter and margarine	no more than 1 tablespoon daily
Red meat	no more than 4 servings per week
Cheese	no more than 1 serving per week
Fried foods	no more than 1 serving per week
Pastries and sweets	no more than 4 servings per week

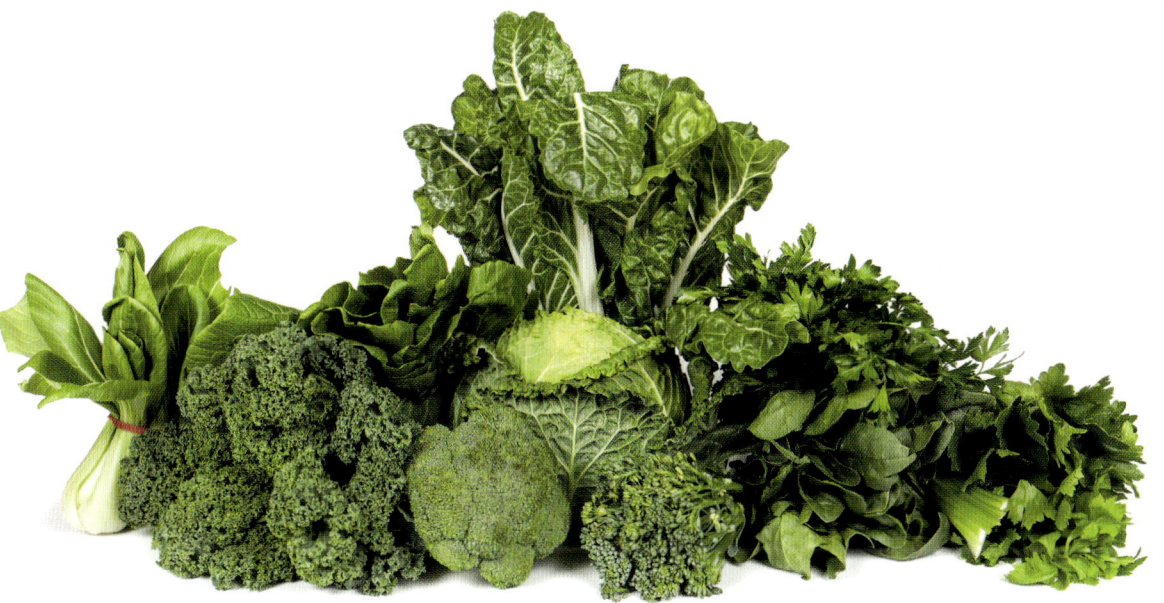

Let's look in a little more detail into why those foods are selected.

Green leafy vegetables like kale, spinach, collard greens, and lettuce have been shown to lower the risk of dementia and cognitive decline. Green leafy vegetables are packed with brain-boosting nutrients like folate, vitamin E, carotenoids, and flavonoids. Aim for at least six servings per week. Ideally, you should eat at least one leafy green vegetable and one other vegetable each day. Kale is also a phenomenal source of readily absorbed calcium, a mineral that is vital to warding off osteoporosis and may help keep blood pressure in a healthy range.

Colorful, non-starchy vegetables are low in calories but high in beneficial nutrients. Try including carrots, beets, broccoli, bell peppers, okra, Brussels sprouts, radishes, and tomatoes in your diet for better brain health.

All **berries** are packed with antioxidants, vitamins, and fiber. But blueberries and strawberries may have special brain benefits. Eat berries at least twice per week for optimal brain health. Strawberries pack plenty of potassium, an essential mineral that helps the body maintain a healthy blood pressure and so may help prevent strokes.

Legumes (such as black beans, pinto beans, kidney beans, and soybeans) and lentils are among the healthiest foods on the planet. They're packed with filling fiber, protein, and B vitamins, which are important for brain health. Their protein content makes them a perfect, nearly fat-free meat alternative. Aim for at least four servings per week. For people who don't eat much (or any) red meat, lentils make an excellent substitute as a source of iron, the mineral essential for carrying oxygen to the body's cells.

Walnuts outmatch other nuts in providing omega-3 fats, which research indicates can promote better brain function, protect the heart and blood vessels from disease, and fight inflammation.

While **nuts** are high in calories and fat, they're also loaded with vitamin E, known for its brain-boosting qualities. Other benefits include healthy fats, protein, and fiber. Choose dry-roasted or raw, unsalted nuts without the extra sodium and sweeteners. Substitute a handful of nuts for processed snacks like chips or pastries. Aim for five servings per week.

Whole grains are rich in vitamins and minerals like magnesium, B vitamins, chromium, iron, and folate. Choose whole grains that are minimally processed. Bulgur wheat, brown rice, quinoa, oatmeal, and whole-grain breads and pastas are great options for the MIND diet. Try to get three servings of whole grains per day.

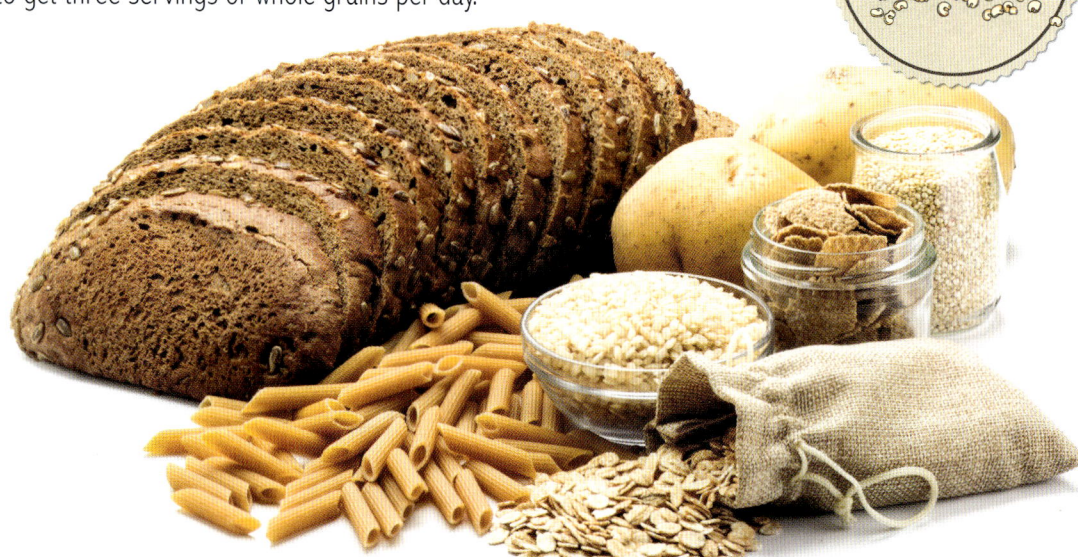

Poultry is a leaner source of protein with more brain benefits than red meat. Eat chicken or turkey at least twice a week. Consume red meat such as beef, pork, and lamb no more than three times per week.

Fish provides quality protein on par with meat but generally contains less total and saturated fat than even the leanest cuts of beef or chicken. What's more, fish contains high levels of omega-3 fatty acids, which have been linked to an amazing array of health benefits, from preventing heart disease and reducing inflammation to improving memory. Excellent sources of omega-3 fatty acids include salmon, mackerel, sardines, anchovies, trout, albacore tuna, bass, and halibut.

Olive oil is a Mediterranean diet staple that has found a home in the MIND diet as well. All oils contain fats, but olive oil is considered healthy because it's mostly made up of heart-healthy monounsaturated fats, with only a small amount of polyunsaturated fat and saturated fat. Extra virgin and virgin olive oils are also rich in flavonoids—antioxidant phytonutrients that help protect cells from damage that can lead to heart disease and cancer.

What About Vegetarianism?

Many people turn to vegetarianism or veganism for ethical reasons related to religion, animal welfare, or care for the environment. Others may turn to vegetarianism and vegan for health reasons, because a plant-based diet can be wonderfully heart-healthy. One meta-analysis of eight observational studies found that vegetarian and vegan diets were associated with a 30 percent reduction risk of mortality caused by ischemic heart disease.

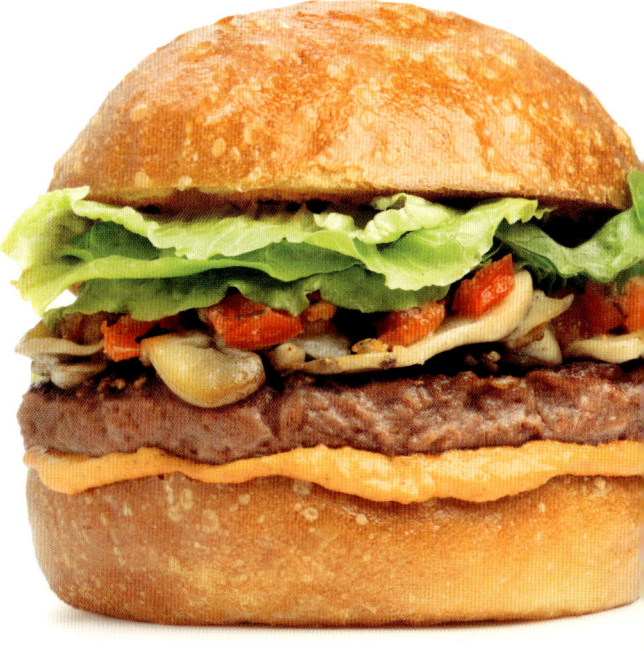

Of course, not every food or diet that is animal-free is healthy by default. A donut may be made without using any animal by-products, but it may also contain a lot of saturated fat and added sugars. If you buy processed vegetarian products such as veggie burgers, you should still check their nutritional labels for their fat, saturated fat, and sodium levels. By and large, though, a vegetarian diet will be full of nutrient-dense plant foods that offer lots of fiber, vitamins, minerals, and antioxidants that are supportive of brain and heart health. Vegetarian diets tend to have lower levels of saturated fat than omnivorous diets—and, of course, plant matter is cholesterol free.

A number of studies have shown better health outcomes, particular in terms of heart disease, by followers of vegetarian diets. A study that followed about 48,000 people in Great Britain for close to twenty years found that those who didn't eat meat had a 20 percent lower risk for coronary artery disease, though it also found that they had a higher risk for a particular kind of stroke, a hemorrhagic stroke. This may be related to lower B12 levels, but no one is really sure why. However, in absolute numbers, more people benefited from their reduction of heart disease risk than were affected by the stroke risk. (In that study pescatarians, who eat fish but not other forms of meat, seemed to get much of the benefit of a heart-healthy eating pattern without any additional stroke risk.)

Plant-based diets have also been shown to be associated with a lower risk of cognitive decline, although in some studies diets referred to as "plant-based" allow for some fish or meat.

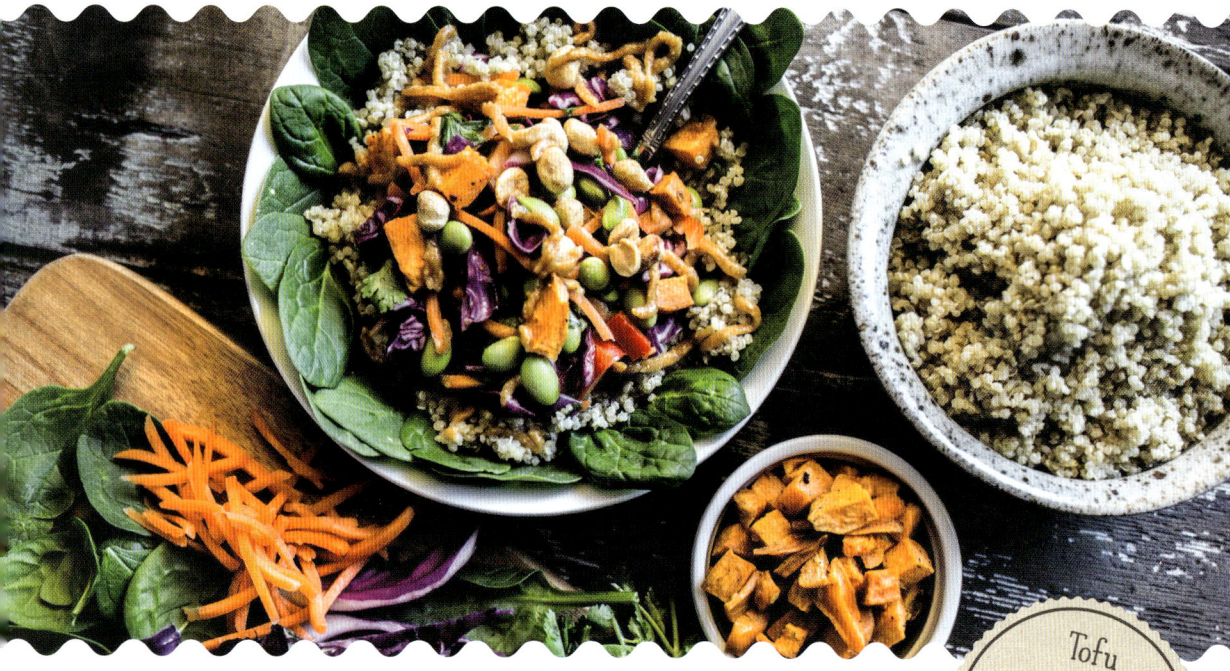

GETTING ALL YOUR NUTRIENTS

While there are some nutrients that are more easily found in animal products, vegetarians can build a well-rounded diet that delivers all their nutritional needs.

Protein: There are a lot of great sources of vegetable protein. Many sources of vegetable protein are not "complete," meaning they don't have all nine essential amino acids. At one point people thought that a vegetarian should "combine" two forms of protein in the same meal in order to get a complete protein source. For example, hummus paired with pita, or rice with beans, were seen as delivering a complete protein. However, the current consensus is that as long as you're eating a varied diet throughout the day, you don't need to sweat the details about any given meal.

The body can only absorb so much protein in one meal; it's recommended that rather than having one protein-heavy meal a day, you space smaller amounts throughout the day.

Good sources of vegetarian protein include soy products such as tofu, tempeh, and edamame; lentils; chickpeas; nuts; an ancient grain called amaranth; quinoa; beans; and seeds such as chia and hemp seeds.

Calcium: Many vegetarians get their calcium from dairy products. Vegan sources of calcium include soy foods; beans, in particular winged, white, navy, and black beans; some nuts, especially almonds; seeds including chia and sesame seeds; and dark leafy greens. While spinach has calcium, it also contains substances called oxalates that prevent absorption. Boiling as a cooking method helps reduce oxalates. Kale and broccoli both have lower oxalate levels than spinach and Swiss chard.

Vitamin B12: Vitamin B12 is found easily in animal products. Plant-based sources are a little more scarce. Vegetarians who still eat dairy and eggs will generally not have any problems. Vegans may turn to fortified foods like fortified breakfast cereals and a substance called nutritional yeast, or "nooch." This powdered yeast is often fortified with not only B12 but also vitamins like riboflavin, folate, and vitamin B6. It has a rich, unami flavor and can be added to casseroles and stews.

Kale

Iron: Non-heme, or plant-based, sources of iron include dried beans and legumes, nuts, seeds, and whole grains. Eating plenty of vitamin C helps you better absorb the iron.

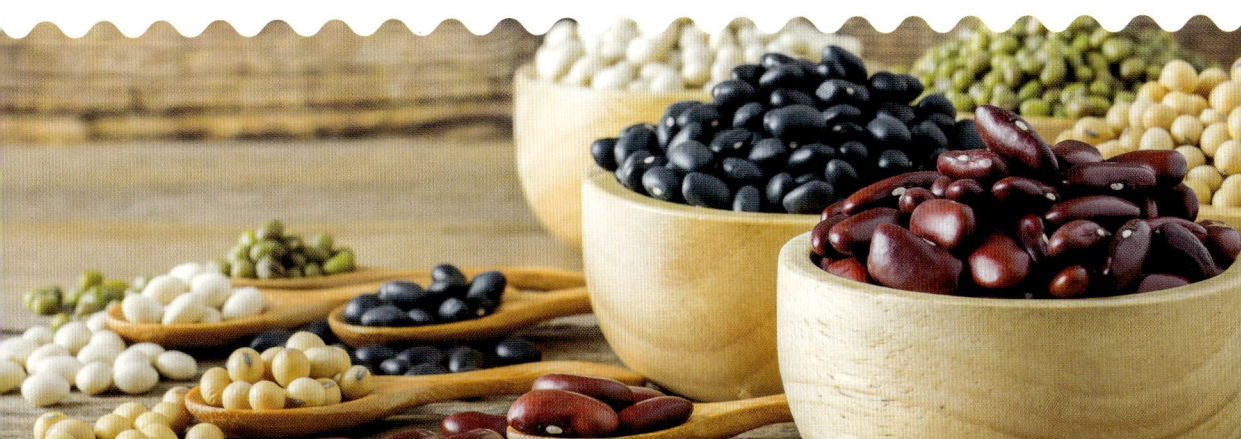

ALLERGIES

Allergies can be called a haywire response of the immune system. Normally, the immune system guards against intruders it considers harmful to the body, such as certain viruses and bacteria. That's its job. However, in allergic people, the immune system goes a bit bonkers. It overreacts when you breathe, ingest, or touch a harmless substance. The benign culprits triggering the overreaction, such as dust, pet dander, and pollen, are called allergens.

The body's first line of defense against invaders includes the nose, mouth, eyes, lungs, and stomach. When the immune system reacts to an allergen, these body parts make great battlegrounds.

Symptoms include runny nose; sneezing; watery, swollen, or red eyes; nasal congestion; wheezing; shortness of breath; a tight feeling in the chest; difficulty breathing; coughing; diarrhea; nausea; headache; fatigue; and a general feeling of misery. Symptoms can occur alone or in combination.

FOODS TO BOOST THAT IMMUNE SYSTEM

An allergy-sufferer's hardworking immune system may increase demands for certain nutrients, both to protect the body and to help rebuild defenses. Be sure your diet includes the following vitamins and minerals:

- Vitamin A. If you eat a well-balanced diet, you should have an ample supply.
- Vitamin B complex. B vitamins are found in almost every food, but the best sources are from fresh vegetables and meats.
- Vitamin C. Citrus fruits are high in vitamin C.
- Vitamin E. High amounts are found in vegetable oils, nuts, and seeds. Moderate amounts are in avocados, asparagus, mangoes, apples, and sweet potatoes.
- Iron. The best sources are meats, oysters, whole grains (including hot cereals), beans, and green vegetables.

- Selenium. Find this mineral in meats, seafood, and whole grains.
- Zinc. Meats, oysters, dairy products, and some beans have good amounts of zinc.

WHAT CAUSES ALLERGIES?

Blame your genes. The tendency to become allergic is inherited, and allergies typically develop before age 30. What you become allergic to is based on what substances you are exposed to and how often you are exposed to them. Generally, the more you are exposed to an allergen, the more likely it is to trigger a reaction.

Unfortunately, there is no cure for allergies. But there are ways to ease your long-suffering sinuses and skin, both in the short term and the long term.

KITCHEN CURES

BASIL. To help ease an allergic reaction or hives, try dousing the skin with basil tea, a traditional Chinese folk remedy. Basil contains high amounts of an anti-allergic compound called caffeic acid. Place 1 ounce dried basil leaves into 1 quart boiling water. Cover and let cool to room temperature. Use the tea as a rinse as often as needed.

MILK. Milk does the body good, especially when it comes to hives. Wet a cloth with cold milk and lay it on the affected area for 10 to 15 minutes. When it comes to drinking, though, pass up the milk. When allergies act up, skip that extra-large, whole-milk latte since dairy products thicken mucus.

TO MAKE MINT TEA:
Place ½ ounce dried mint leaves in a 1-quart jar. Fill two-thirds of the jar with boiling water and steep for five minutes (inhale the steam). Let cool, strain, sweeten if desired, and drink.

TEA. Allergy sufferers throughout the centuries have turned to hot tea to provide relief for clogged-up noses and irritated mucous membranes. One of the best for symptom relief is mint tea, which has been used by the Chinese to treat allergies since the seventh century. Mint's benefits extend well beyond its delicious smell. Mint's essential oils act as a decongestant, and substances within the mint contain anti-inflammatory and mild antibacterial constituents.

WASABI. If you're a hay fever sufferer and sushi lover combined, this remedy will please. Wasabi, that pale-green, fiery condiment served alongside California rolls, is a member of the horseradish family. Anyone who has taken too big a dollop of wasabi or plain old horseradish knows how it makes sinuses and tear ducts spring into action. That's because allyl isothiocyanate, a constituent in wasabi, promotes phlegm flow and has antiasthmatic properties. The tastiest way to get in those allyl isothiocyanates is by slathering horseradish on your sandwich or plopping wasabi onto your favorite sushi. The last, harder-to-swallow option is to purchase grated horseradish and take ¼ teaspoon during an allergy attack.

ALZHEIMER'S DISEASE

Alzheimer's disease (AD) is everyone's worst nightmare. Most diseases destroy either a physical or a mental function. Alzheimer's seizes both, slowly and steadily destroying memory, logical thought, and language. Simple tasks—how to eat or comb hair—are forgotten. AD is one of a group of brain disorders called dementia, which are progressive degenerative brain syndromes that affect memory, thinking, behavior, and emotion. Alzheimer's is the most common cause of dementia: Between 50 and 60 percent of all cases of dementia can be attributed to Alzheimer's.

Early symptoms include difficulty remembering names, places, or faces and trouble recalling things that just happened. Personality changes and confusion when driving a car or handling money are also early symptoms. Eventually mild forgetfulness progresses to problems in comprehension, speaking, reading, and writing. Physical breakdown occurs, too, partly because tasks such as eating and drinking are simply forgotten or too difficult to accomplish.

Since we don't know what causes AD, we also do not yet have a cure for it. However, the picture is not as bleak as it was a decade ago. Research is turning up some remedies that can help alleviate symptoms as well as slow the advancement of the disease. And the good news is that many of these can be found right in your kitchen.

KITCHEN CURES

ALMOND EXTRACT. This contains vitamin E. Try baking some almond cookies.

BLUEBERRIES. Evidence suggests they contain an antioxidant that may slow down age-related motor changes, such as those seen in Alzheimer's.

CARROTS. These are loaded with beta-carotene, which is a memory booster. Carrot and beet juice are good for the memory, too. So are okra and spinach.

CITRUS FRUITS. These fruits are loaded with vitamin C, which is believed to help protect brain nerves. Berries and some vegetables, including peppers, sweet potatoes, and green leafy vegetables, are also rich sources of vitamin C.

EGGS. It doesn't matter how you eat them. Eggs are loaded with vitamin A, which may protect brain cells and enhance brain function. Other vitamin A-rich foods include liver, spinach, milk, squash, and peaches.

FISH. Fatty acids, which AD sufferers often lack, are important in keeping those brain nerves healthy. Fish are high in fatty acids (that's why they're often called "brain food"), so it's a good idea to eat fish several times a week. Good choices include salmon, mackerel, sardines, and anchovies.

GINGER. This spice can stimulate a poor appetite. Try some ginger tea or gingersnaps, or chop up some fresh ginger and mix it with a little lime juice and a pinch of rock salt, then chew. It will not only increase appetite but thirst, too.

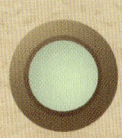
Orange

EASY EATING

Using utensils can become difficult for people with Alzheimer's, so solve the problem by offering finger foods. Keep them simple, handy, and nutritious.

Some suggestions:

- Fortified breads
- Peanut butter sandwich
- Easy to grab fruits, such as bananas, apricots (especially dried apricots, which are high in potassium), peeled apple wedges (apple peels can cause choking), carrots, and celery sticks
- Chocolate-covered almonds or almond M&Ms. Almonds are rich in vitamin E, which may delay the progression of AD. Two ounces of almonds a day supplies the recommended amount of vitamin E.

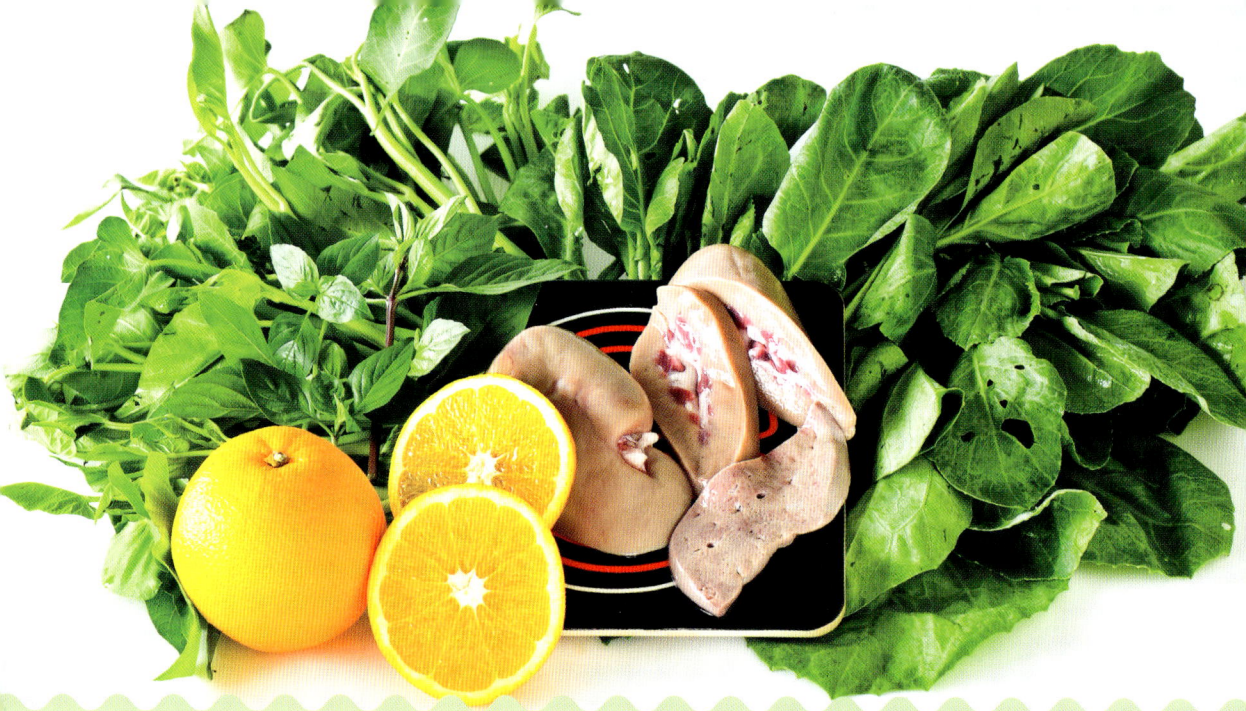

GREEN LEAFY VEGETABLES. These are high in folic acid, which may stimulate cognitive function. Other good sources of folic acid include beets, black-eyed peas and other legumes, Brussels sprouts, and whole-grain foods.

LEMON OIL. Steep a few drops of lemon or peppermint oil in hot water, then inhale. These are aromatherapy stimulants; they can perk up those suffering typical AD symptoms such as lethargy or depression.

MEAL SUPPLEMENTS. These meal-in-a-can beverages are easy to drink, and they're fortified with vitamins and minerals.

ORANGE JUICE. This is another way to up your vitamin C intake, but don't combine it with buffered aspirin. The two, taken together, form aluminum citrate, which is absorbed into the body five times faster than normal aluminum.

RED VEGETABLES. Research from the Netherlands suggests that people who eat large amounts of dark red, yellow, and green vegetables may reduce their risk of dementia by 25 percent.

SAGE. For depression associated with AD, drink a tea made with ½ teaspoon sage and ¼ teaspoon basil steeped in 1 cup hot water twice a day.

SEEDS. Pumpkin, sesame, and sunflower seeds are packed with essential fatty acids necessary for brain function.

SESAME OIL. Depression associated with AD may be relieved with nose drops of warmed sesame oil. Use about 3 drops per nostril, twice a day.

SOY PRODUCTS. Studies suggest that isoflavones found in soy protein may protect postmenopausal women from AD. Try these: soy milk over cereal, soy meat substitutes, tofu frozen treats. And substitute tofu for ricotta or cream cheese in recipes. Dietary guidelines suggest 20 to 25 grams soy protein a day.

TURMERIC. Curcumin, an antioxidant and anti-inflammatory compound in this spice, has been found to reduce the number of plaques in the brain of mice and thus may slow the progression of Alzheimer's.

WHEAT GERM OR POWDERED MILK. Add to foods for extra protein.

Turmeric

DO'S & DON'TS FOR CAREGIVERS

- Don't serve foods with pits or bones.
- Always check food temperature. Hot and cold sensations can be numbed in people with AD, but they still can get burned.
- Don't serve foods with a mixture of textures. They may be hard to swallow.
- Serve foods that require little chewing, such as soups, ground meat, and applesauce.
- Serve several smaller meals instead of three main meals.
- Select favorite foods, especially if the appetite is poor. And keep in mind that as the disease progresses, food preferences may change.
- Play music at meals. Mealtimes can be stressful and music is relaxing. Choose songs from the patient's youth or that hold a special memory.

BANANA BASICS

It's one of nature's true miracles, and for those with Alzheimer's, it's a nutritional miracle. One of the most common problems plaguing people with AD is low fluid intake. Those with the disease simply forget to drink, or they choose not to in order to avoid bathroom emergencies and accidents. The result is dehydration, which can cause a loss of potassium, which in turn, contributes to confusion. The simple solution for restoring essential potassium to the body is to force fluids—water or sports drinks with potassium—but that's often easier said than done. Bananas are a great source of fast energy. Very ripe bananas are loaded with sugar, about 23 grams, which is digested quickly and easily, then converted into energy. Bananas are easy to chew and swallow, which can be very important in AD since these functions may become impaired.

ANEMIA

Anemia is a condition in which your red blood cell count is so low that it can't carry enough oxygen to all parts of your body. Not having enough oxygen in the blood is like trying to drive a car with no oil. Your car may run for a while, but you'll soon end up with a burned-out engine. In the same way that oil nourishes your car's engine, oxygen provides needed nourishment for your body's tissues (organs, muscles, etc.), and if they aren't getting enough of that vital sustenance, you'll start feeling weak and tired. A short climb up the stairs will leave you breathless, and even a couple days of rest won't perk you up. If that describes how you feel, check with your doctor. If you do have anemia, you should take action as soon as possible. And you need to be sure you don't have a more serious condition.

ANATOMY OF ANEMIA

Your red blood cells are the delivery trucks of the body. They carry oxygen throughout your blood vessels and capillaries to feed tissues. Hemoglobin, the primary component of red blood cells, is a complex molecule and is the oxygen carrier of the red blood cell.

The body works very hard to ensure that it produces enough red blood cells to successfully carry oxygen but not too many, which can cause the blood to get too thick. Red blood cells live only 90 to 120 days. The liver and spleen get rid of the old cells, though the iron in the cells is recycled and sent back to the marrow to produce new cells.

When you're diagnosed with anemia it usually means your red blood cell count is abnormally low, so it can't carry enough oxygen to all parts of your body, or that there is a reduction in the hemoglobin content of your red blood cells. Anemia is not a disease in itself but instead is considered a condition. However, this condition can be a symptom of a more serious illness. That's why it's always important to check with your doctor if you think you may be anemic.

IRON'S ABSORPTION EQUATION

You may not be absorbing as much iron from your foods as you think. How much you absorb is dependent on two primary factors: what kind of iron is in the food and what other nutrients the food contains. There are two types of iron, heme and non-heme. Heme, found primarily in foods of animal origin, is much more easily absorbed than non-heme iron, which is found primarily in plant products. But if you eat a vitamin C-rich food or a food rich in heme iron with your non-heme iron food, your body will take in more iron.

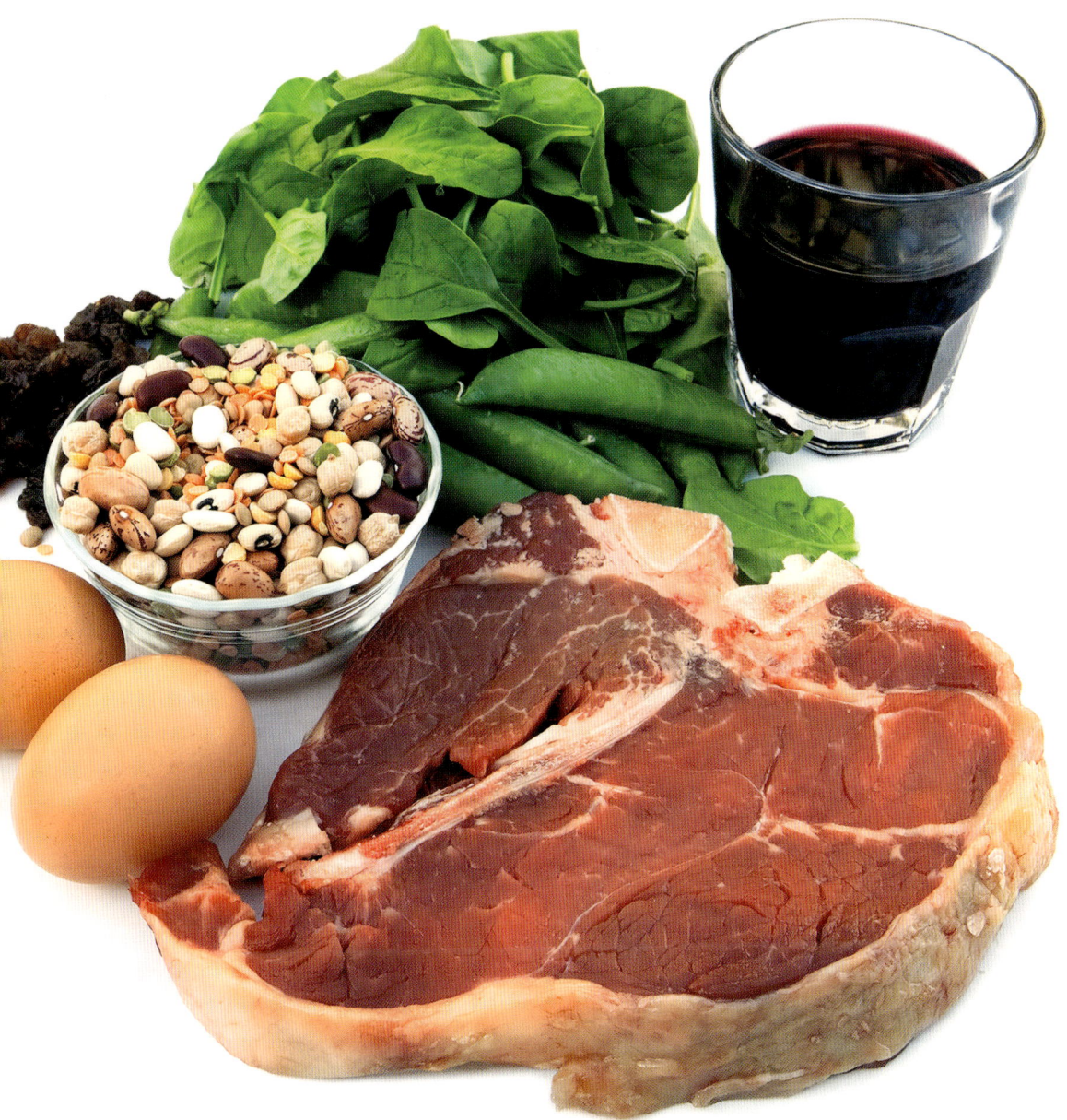

Here's a guide to top iron sources:

- Sources of mostly heme iron: beef liver, lean sirloin, lean ground beef, skinless chicken, pork
- Sources of non-heme iron: fortified breakfast cereal, pumpkin seeds, bran, spinach
- Sources of vitamin B12: salmon, beef tenderloin, yogurt, shrimp
- Sources of folic acid: spinach, navy beans, wheat germ, avocado, orange

KITCHEN CURES

BLACKSTRAP MOLASSES. Consider covering that waffle or those pancakes in a little molasses. Blackstrap molasses has long been known to be a nutritional powerhouse. Containing 3.5 mg of iron per tablespoon, blackstrap molasses has been used in folk medicine as a "blood builder" for centuries.

DRY CEREAL. Fix yourself a bowl of your favorite cereal (go for one without the sugar and the cartoon characters on the box), and you'll be waging a battle against anemia. These days many cereals are fortified with a nutrient punch of iron, vitamin B12, and folic acid. Check the label for amounts per serving, pour some milk over your flakes, and dig in.

BEEF LIVER. Beef liver is rich in iron and all the B vitamins (including B12 and folic acid). In fact, beef liver contains more iron per serving—5.8 mg per 3 ounces—than any other food. Other animal sources of iron include eggs, cheese, fish, lean sirloin, lean ground beef, and chicken.

BEETS. Beets are rich in folic acid, as well as many other nutrients, such as fiber and potassium. The best way to prepare beets is to nuke 'em in the microwave. Keep the skin on when cooking, but peel before eating. The most nutrient-dense part of the beet is right under the skin.

SPINACH. Green leafy vegetables contain loads of iron and folic acid. We're talking dark and green, so choose your leaves carefully. Iceberg lettuce is mostly water and is of little nutritive value. Spinach, on the other hand, has 3.2 mg of iron and 130 mcg of folic acid per ½ cup.

DO'S AND DON'TS

- If you're a vegetarian or have cut way down on your intake of meats, milk, and eggs, be sure that you're getting adequate amounts of iron and vitamin B12 in your diet. With such a diet, you are at greater risk for nutritional deficiency anemias because iron from plant sources isn't absorbed as well as iron from animal sources and because vitamin B12 is found almost exclusively in animal foods.

- Eat foods rich in vitamin C at the same time that you eat whole grains, spinach, and legumes, in order to increase absorption of the iron they contain.

- If you drink coffee or tea, do so between meals rather than with meals, because the caffeine in these beverages reduces iron absorption.

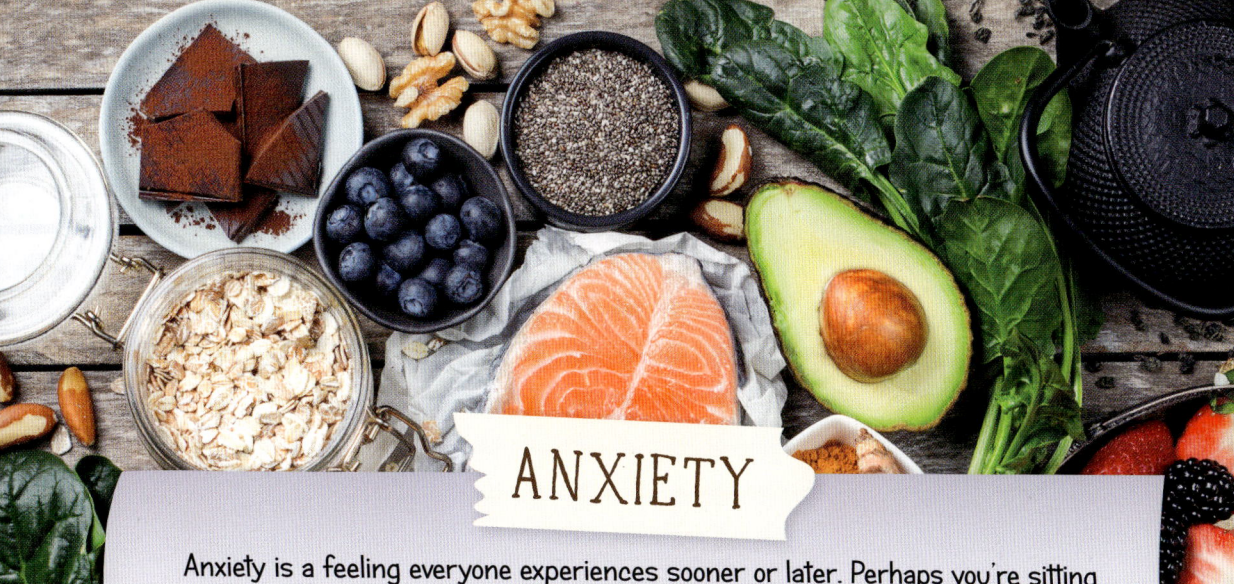

ANXIETY

Anxiety is a feeling everyone experiences sooner or later. Perhaps you're sitting in the waiting room, anticipating the horse-size needle your doctor has waiting for you on the other side of the door. Or you've spent all day cooking but the look on your mother-in-law's face says your best efforts were wasted. Or you really hate your job. These very different experiences can bring on anxiety and its typical symptoms: heart palpitations, a sense of impending doom, inability to concentrate, muscle tension, dry mouth, sweating, a queasy, jittery feeling in the pit of the stomach, and hyperventilation.

Anxiety can be short- or long-lived, depending on its source. The more long lasting the anxiety, the more additional symptoms you will experience. If your anxiety is a reaction to a single, isolated event—the shot the doctor is about to give you—your anxiety level will decrease and your symptoms will disappear after the event. If your anxiety is from friction between you and your mother-in-law, you're likely to experience anxiety for a period of time before and after you see her. In this case, the symptom list may have grown to include diarrhea or constipation and irritability.

Then there's that job, a source of anxiety that never leaves you. You dread getting up in the morning because you have to go to work, dread going to bed at night because when you wake up you have to go to work, dread the weekend because when it's over you'll have to go to work. When the source of your anxiety is ever-present, you can probably add the following to the list of symptoms: chest pain, over- or under-eating, insomnia, loss of sex drive.

Mild anxiety can be often treated successfully at home with a little calming music, a little quiet time, and some soothing remedies from the kitchen.

KITCHEN CURES

ALMONDS. Soak 10 raw almonds overnight in water to soften, then peel off the skins. Put almonds in blender with 1 cup warm milk, a pinch of ginger, and a pinch of nutmeg. Drink at night to relax you before going to bed.

ORANGE. The aroma of an orange is known to reduce anxiety. All you have to do to get the benefits is peel an orange and inhale. You can also drop the peel into a small pan or potpourri burner. Cover with water and simmer. When heated, the orange peel will release its fragrant and calming oil.

ORANGE JUICE. For a "giddyap" heart rate associated with anxiety, stir 1 teaspoon honey, and a pinch of nutmeg into 1 cup orange juice and drink.

TIPS ON CUTTING THE CAFFEINE

Because caffeine can cause anxiety, and caffeine addiction symptoms mimic anxiety, this good-morning pick-me-up is at the head of the no-no list. But cutting it out all at once can cause withdrawal symptoms, including anxiety, irritability, headache, and fatigue.

To stop, cut back gradually until you are caffeine free and have no withdrawal symptoms. If you do experience withdrawal symptoms, especially as you near the end of all caffeine consumption, continue drinking 1 cup of a caffeinated beverage daily, then gradually cut back on that.

GETTING YOUR VITAMINS

A deficiency in the B vitamins niacin and thiamin, as well as in omega-3 fatty acids and calcium, can contribute to anxiety. Here are some foods you might include more frequently in your diet if you're experiencing an uptick in anxiety.

Niacin-rich Foods

- Liver
- Red meats
- Fish
- Yeast extracts
- Peanuts
- Legumes
- Dried fruits

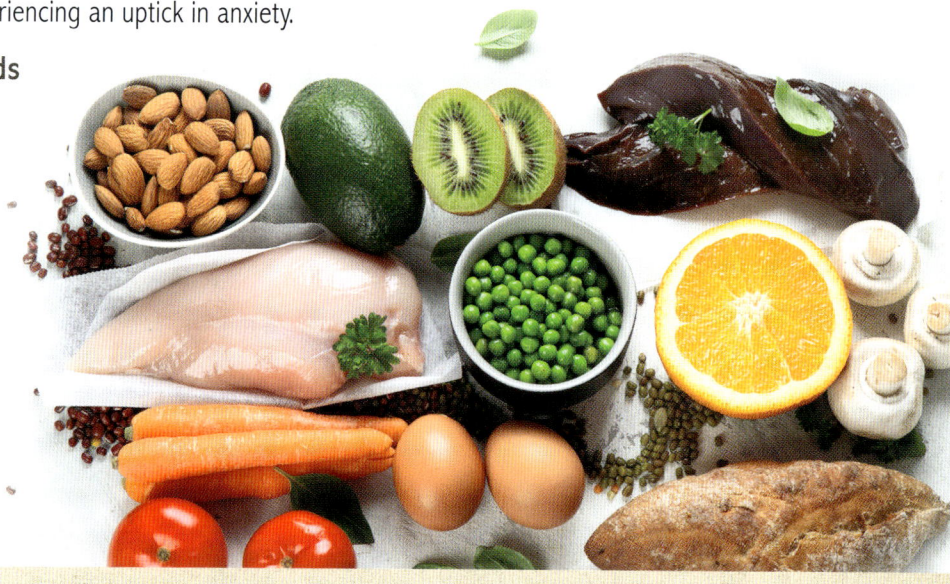

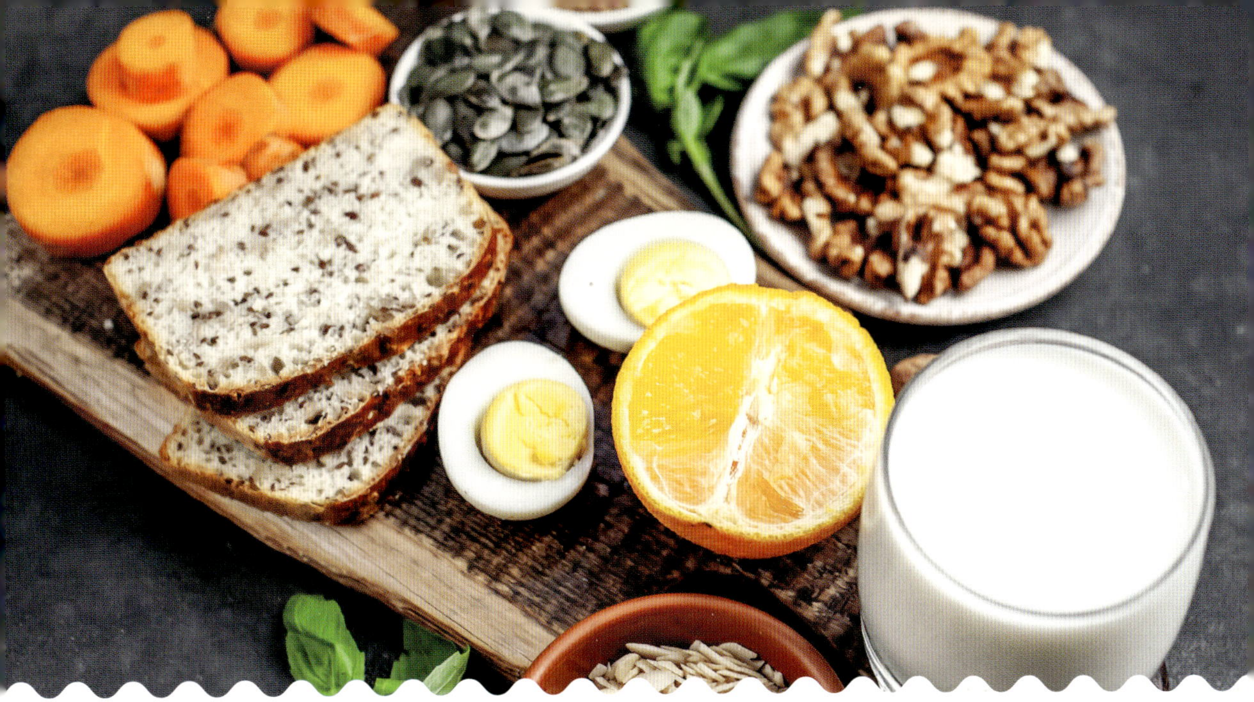

Thiamin-rich Foods

- Whole-wheat products
- Legumes
- Wheat germ
- Bran
- Eggs
- Whole-grain rice

Calcium-rich Foods

- Almonds
- Broccoli
- Cottage cheese
- Milk
- Salmon
- Yogurt

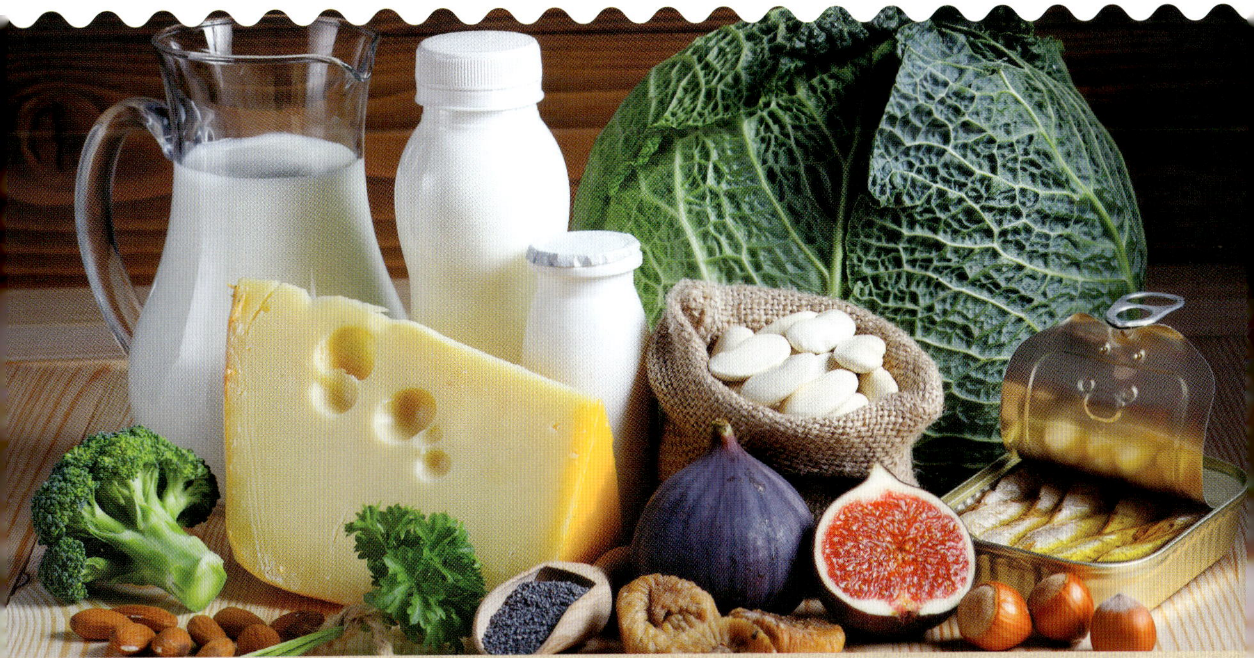

ARTHRITIS

Arthritis means inflammation of the joints. To the millions of Americans afflicted by one of the 100 varieties of arthritis, every day can be painful. The two most prevalent forms of arthritis are osteoarthritis and rheumatoid arthritis.

Osteoarthritis (OA), the most common form, is the result of joint cartilage wearing down over time. When the durable, elastic tissue is gone, bones rub directly against one another. This causes stiffness and dull pain in the weight-bearing joints (hips, knees, and spine) and in the hands. The elderly are most susceptible to OA, but athletes and those in jobs requiring repetitive movements are also very vulnerable.

Rheumatoid arthritis (RA) is the inflammation of the joint lining. The cause is unknown, but it is thought that the symptoms are the result of the body turning against itself. Symptoms of RA vary from individual to individual. In its mildest form, it causes minor joint discomfort. More often, however, the inflammation causes painful, stiff, swollen joints, and in prolonged cases, severe joint damage. Unlike OA, whose symptoms are joint-specific, RA tends to cause body-wide symptoms such as fatigue, fever, and weight loss.

There is no cure for arthritis, but many kitchen-crafted remedies can help ease the pain.

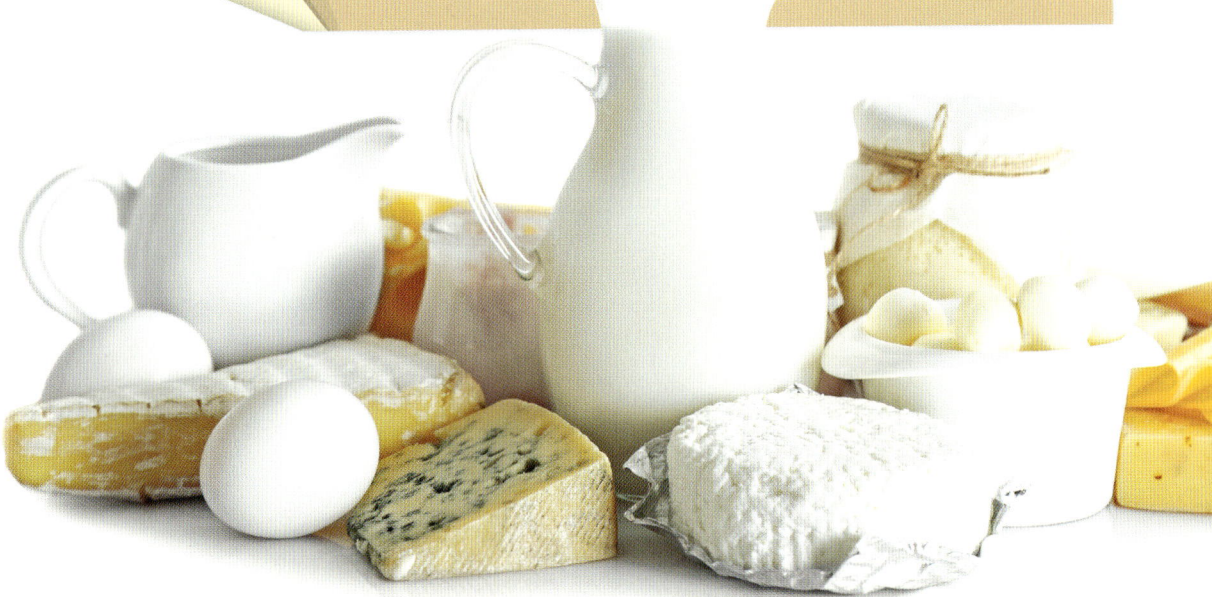

KITCHEN CURES

DAIRY PRODUCTS. Some medicines used to treat arthritis can lead to a loss of calcium from the bones, resulting in osteoporosis. To counteract this effect (and to keep healthy in general) make sure you get enough calcium in your diet. A cup of low-fat yogurt, for instance, supplies 300 to 400 mg calcium—about one-third of your daily requirement. Calcium-fortified orange juice will also help you meet your daily calcium needs.

GAMMA LINOLENIC ACID. Recent research suggests that high doses of an omega-6 essential fatty acid, known as gamma linolenic acid (GLA), can help reduce joint inflammation. You'll find GLA in some plant seed oils, such as evening primrose and borage, and in black currants. Research also indicates that the benefits of GLA may be enhanced by supplementation with omega-3 fatty acids, which are plentiful in cold-water fish. You can also take GLA supplements; 1,800 mg a day is recommended for rheumatoid arthritis.

TRACK WHAT WORKS

Decreasing arthritis pain and stiffness may be as easy as eliminating certain foods from your refrigerator and, thus, from your diet. However, the deduction process is a bit difficult, requiring time and observation. There are no set guidelines for this remedy. Rather, it is intuitive. Do you ache more after eating a certain food? Keep a food diary, record what you've eliminated from your diet that week, and rate your discomfort level. There are no guarantees, but you may discover that certain foods contribute to stiffness.

SETTING UP YOUR KITCHEN

Little adjustments in the kitchen itself may make a big difference in protecting arthritic joints from injury or excessive strain.

- Buy kitchen drawer knobs with long, thin handles. These require a looser, less stressful grip.
- More padding, less pain. On tools that require a grip, such as mops and brooms, tape a layer of thin foam rubber around the handles and fasten with tape.
- Use lightweight pots and pans with comfortable handles.
- Utilize a pair of long-handled pinchers (or a gripper) to pick up objects on the floor.
- Transport groceries or heavy items from car to kitchen using a wagon or cart.
- Use loops made of soft, strong fabric to pull the refrigerator and oven doors open without strain.

ASTHMA

Asthma is the number one cause of chronic illness in kids, affecting more than 4.5 million children. Despite this discouraging news, there is reason to be hopeful if you are one of the millions of asthmatics across the country. As the numbers of asthma cases continue to climb, researchers are even more determined to find asthma's causes and develop more effective treatments.

BREATHING BASICS

When you take a breath, the air goes from your mouth or nose to the windpipe (or trachea). It then travels to the lungs. It first enters the lungs through the bronchi, a group of tubes that branch off from the windpipe. The bronchi then branch off into bronchioles. Imagine a car driving from the interstate to a state highway to a country road and you get the picture. Asthma happens when the bronchi and bronchioles come in contact with a foreign invader, or asthma "trigger." There are many different triggers, and each person has his own set. Once a foreign material enters the body, the airways quickly become inflamed, causing the muscles that rest on the outside of the airways to tighten and narrow. This allows a thick mucus to enter the airways. The mucus causes swelling and makes it very difficult to breathe. The classic symptoms of an asthma attack include wheezing, tightening in the chest, dry coughing, and increased heart rate. These are frightening symptoms to experience, and they're also quite alarming for someone to observe.

Though there are many natural ways to help asthma sufferers breathe easier, experts recommend that combining certain natural remedies with prescription anti-inflammatories and bronchodilators are your best bet to attack your asthma.

KITCHEN CURES

COFFEE. The caffeine in regular coffee can help prevent and treat asthma attacks. Researchers have found that regular coffee drinkers have one-third fewer asthma symptoms than those who don't drink the hot stuff. And caffeine has bronchodilating effects. In fact, caffeine was one of the main anti-asthmatic drugs during the nineteenth century. Don't load up on java, though. Three cups a day will provide the maximum benefit.

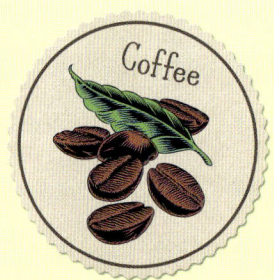

CHILI PEPPERS. Hot foods such as chili peppers open up airways. Experts believe this happens because peppers stimulate fluids in the mouth, throat, and lungs. The increase in fluids thins out the mucus formed during an asthma attack so it can be coughed up, making breathing easier. Capsaicin, the stuff that makes hot peppers hot, acts as an anti-inflammatory when eaten and a bronchodilator when inhaled in small doses.

ONIONS. Onions are loaded with anti-inflammatory properties. Studies have shown that these properties can reduce the constriction of the airways in an asthma attack. Use cooked onions, as raw onions are generally too irritating.

ORANGE JUICE. Vitamin C is the main antioxidant in the lining of the bronchi and bronchioles. Research discovered that people with asthma had low levels of vitamin C and that eating foods that had at least 300 mg of vitamin C a day—equivalent to about 3 glasses of orange juice—cut wheezing by 30 percent. Other foods high in vitamin C include red bell pepper, papaya, broccoli, blueberries, and strawberries.

SALMON. Fatty fish such as sardines, salmon, mackerel, and tuna contain omega-3 fatty acids. These fatty acids seem to help the lungs react better to irritants in people who have asthma and may even help prevent asthma in people who have never had an attack. Studies have found that kids who eat fish more than once a week have one-third the chance of getting asthma as children who don't eat fish. And researchers discovered that people who took fish oil supplements, equivalent to eating 8 ounces of mackerel a day, increased their body's ability to avoid a severe asthma attack by 50 percent.

FOODS TO AVOID

Some asthma sufferers are particularly sensitive to the chemical preservatives sulfites. Sulfites are found in many kinds of foods and beverages. If you have a question about a food, check out the label. Sulfites will probably be listed among the ingredients. Here are some common foods with high concentrations of sulfites:

- Wine
- Lemon juice
- Dried fruits
- Fresh shrimp
- Instant potatoes
- Canned veggies
- Fruit topping
- Molasses
- Wine vinegar
- Corn syrup
- Pizza dough
- Grapes
- Beer
- Instant tea

BACK PAIN

People are bad to their backs, crouching over keyboards for eight hours, struggling to lift heavy objects, or quickly transforming themselves from sedentary office workers to weekend warriors. Whatever the action, the back often can't handle such stress, and it reacts with pain.

Almost everyone will experience back pain once in their life. Lower back pain has many causes, including common muscle strain and more serious problems with the bones in the spine (vertebrae) and the disks of shock-absorbing material that separate them. Why is the lower back such a glutton for punishment? Unlike the upper back, it isn't supported by the rib cage, and many people don't exercise the back and the supporting abdominal muscles as they should.

Back pain remedies rely primarily on rest, strengthening and stretching exercises, and modification of daily routine. However, the kitchen shelves do hold a few ingredients that can help get that back back into shape.

KITCHEN CURES

CHAMOMILE TEA. Daily stress can turn back muscles into a knot. Luckily, chamomile tea offers some calming relief to soothe tense muscle tissue. During a break or after work, treat yourself to a steaming mug. Steep 1 tablespoon chamomile flowers in 1 cup boiling water for 15 minutes. Or, you can use a prepackaged chamomile tea. Drink 1 to 3 cups a day.

Warning! Chamomile contains allergy-inducing proteins related to ragweed pollen. Ask your doctor about drinking chamomile if you are allergic to ragweed. Packaged tea may be safer to drink than tea made from the flowers. Your doctor can advise you.

GINGER ROOT. Fragrant ginger root has long been known to cure nausea, but back pain, too? Ginger does contain anti-inflammatory compounds, including some with mild aspirinlike effects. When your back aches, cut a 1- to 2-inch fresh ginger root into slices and place in 1 quart boiling water. Simmer, covered, for 30 minutes on low heat. Cool for 30 minutes. Strain, sweeten with honey (to taste), and drink.

MILK. Bone up on milk. Women especially should take care to include plenty of calcium in their diets. (Older women are at greater risk for developing osteoporosis, the disease of eroding bones.) Calcium helps build strong bones and protect the spine from osteoporosis.

ROSEMARY. Rosemary's leaves are packed with these anti-inflammatory substances: carnosol, oleanolic acid, rosmarinic acid, and ursolic acid, all of which work to ease swollen tissues. To make a pain-relieving tea: Place ½ ounce dried rosemary leaves into 1 quart boiling water. Cover and steep for 30 minutes. Drink 1 cup tea at bedtime and another cup before eating breakfast.

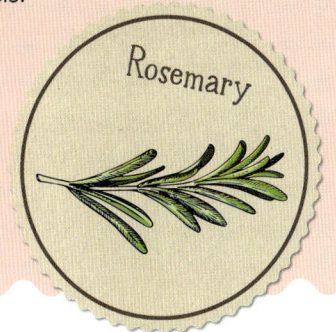

BELCHING

It's not a big deal, not even a medical condition most of the time. It's simply the result of swallowing air. But the air that goes down has to go somewhere, so most of the time it leaves the same way it came in—through the mouth. We all belch. Even the most prim of the proper is not exempt from this oftentimes untimely eruption.

Belching does serve a purpose other than embarrassment, however. It removes gas from the stomach by forcing it up into the esophagus and then on out your mouth. Without this escape device, we'd blow up like a big balloon, not to mention the sharp cramps we'd feel running all the way from our stomach to our throats. So belching is a good thing. And no matter how many good ones we let out during the course of a day, the swallowed air that turns into a burp is only a tiny fraction of the intestinal gas that we all have.

THE CAUSE

Swallowing air, which is called aerophagia, is the primary offender when it comes to producing a belch. We swallow air all the time, especially when we

- Eat and drink
- Talk
- Yawn and sigh
- Breathe through the mouth
- Smoke
- Chew gum or suck on hard candy

Here are some other reasons we belch:

- Belching occurs when we eat because food in the belly displaces the air that was already swallowed and is sitting in the stomach.

- Anxiety is a cause of belching, too. We get nervous, we swallow more air. The more nervous we are, the more air we swallow, and the more we belch. Anxiety belching is usually habitual and subconscious. We swallow air into the esophagus and expel it before it hits the stomach.

- An improper denture fit can cause you to swallow air.

- Drinking carbonated beverages.

- Excessive swallowing due to postnasal drip.

- Although belching is not normally a symptom of illness, some gastrointestinal disorders are accompanied by belching, including gallstones, hiatal hernia, ulcer, and gastritis.

Even with all the conditions belching could potentially indicate, most often belching is simply belching for the sake of letting out unneeded gasses.

Of course, that occasional and inadvertent little burp may slip out, and often at the most embarrassing moment. If its escape is, indeed, occasional, there's nothing to worry about. But if it happens more often than you'd like, you can look to your kitchen for a cure.

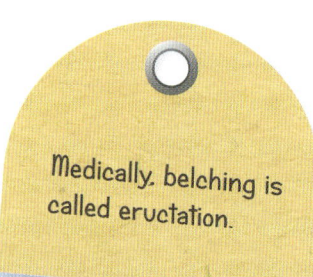

Medically, belching is called eructation.

KITCHEN CURES

CARAWAY. Try some caraway seeds, straight or sprinkled on a salad. They calm the digestive tract.

CUMIN. Roast equal amounts of cumin, fennel, and celery seed. Combine. After you eat, chew well about ½ to 1 teaspoon of the mixture, then chase it down with ⅓ cup of warm water.

DILL SEED TEA. Drop 1 teaspoon dill seeds into 1 cup boiling water, then steep for 15 minutes. Strain, then drink. Try the same with fennel or chamomile.

GINGER. Ginger tea can help relieve the need to belch. Pour 1 cup boiling water over 1 teaspoon freshly grated gingerroot. Steep for 5 minutes, then drink.

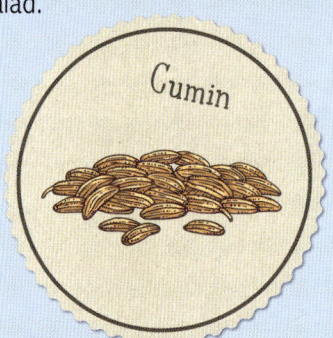

Cumin

LEMON JUICE. This works whether it's fresh or from the bottle. Mix 1 teaspoon lemon juice with ½ teaspoon baking soda in 1 cup cool water. Drink it quickly after meals.

PAPAYA. Most cures for belching aren't found in the fridge. But there is one surefire belch begone in the fruit drawer: papaya! It's full of an enzyme called papain that can get rid of whatever's causing that burp.

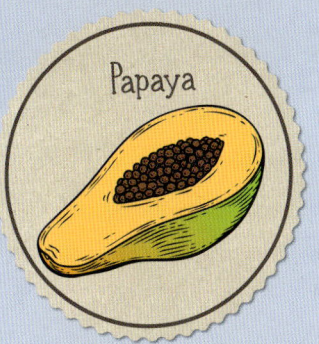
Papaya

PEPPERMINT. Pour 1 cup boiling water over 1 teaspoon dried mint. Steep for five minutes.

YOGURT. Eat some yogurt with live cultures (check the label) every day. It aids digestion.

BRONCHITIS

That nasty cold has been hanging on much longer than it should, and day by day it seems to be getting worse. Your chest hurts, you gurgle when you breathe, and you're coughing so much yellow, green, or grey mucus that your throat is raw. These symptoms are letting you know that your cold has probably turned into a respiratory infection called bronchitis, an inflammation of the little branches and tubes of your windpipe that also makes them swell. No wonder breathing has become such a chore. Your air passages are too puffy to carry air very easily.

Bronchitis is not contagious since it's a secondary infection that develops when your immune system is weakened by a cold or the flu. Under most circumstances, bronchitis will go away on its own once the primary infection is cured. But in those few days when you have it, it can sure be miserable. Here are a few kitchen tips that can relieve some of the symptoms.

Almonds

KITCHEN CURES

ALMONDS. These little cure-all nuts have loads of vitamins and nutrients. Rich in potassium, calcium, and magnesium, almonds are especially known for their healing powers in respiratory illness. So when you're down with bronchitis, eat them in any form, except candy-coated or chocolate-covered. Sliver some almonds and garnish your veggies.

Almonds are also good in a citrus fruit salad for a little added crunch or rubbed in a little honey, coated with cinnamon, and roasted in a 325°F oven for 10 to 25 minutes.

ANISEED. Here's a bronchitis cough reliever that's also said to relieve heartburn. Boil 1 quart water, then add 7 teaspoons aniseed. Simmer until the water is half gone, strain the seeds, and add 4 teaspoons each of honey and glycerine (glycerine is available at the drugstore). Take 2 teaspoons every few hours.

BAY LEAF. Ancient Romans and Greeks loved bay leaves. They believed that this simple herb was the source of happiness, clairvoyance, and artistic inspiration. Whatever the case, it does act as an expectorant and is best taken in tea. To make the tea, tear a leaf (fresh or dried) and steep in 1 cup boiling water. *Warning!* Bay leaf tea should not be used during pregnancy, as it may bring on menstruation. Another bronchitis remedy with bay leaf is to soak some leaves in hot water and apply as a poultice to the chest. Cover with a kitchen towel. As it cools, rewarm.

GINGER. This is a potent expectorant that works well in tea. Steep ½ teaspoon ginger, a pinch of ground cloves, and a pinch of cinnamon in 1 cup boiling water.

HONEY. To relieve the cough that comes from bronchitis, slice an onion into a bowl, then cover with honey. Allow to stand overnight, then remove the onion. Take 1 teaspoon of the honey four times a day.

HORSERADISH. The irritating allyl isothiocyanates (mustard derivatives) in horseradish open up the sinuses. Be careful not to use horseradish if you're having stomach problems, though, because it's too potent. Eat it straight, on a salad, or atop meat. Fresh horseradish is the best choice, but commercial products will work, too. Make sure it's straight horseradish, though. Sandwich spreads with horseradish won't work.

LEMONS. These help rid the respiratory system of bacteria and mucus. Make a cup of lemon tea by grating 1 teaspoon lemon rind and adding it to 1 cup boiling water. Steep for five minutes. Or, you can boil a lemon wedge. Strain into a cup and drink. For a sore throat that comes from coughing, add 1 teaspoon lemon juice to 1 cup warm water and gargle. This helps bring up phlegm.

ONIONS. These are expectorants and help the flow of mucus. Use raw, cooked, baked, in soups and stews, as seasoning, or any which way you like them.

SAVORY. This potent, peppery herb is said to rid the lungs of mucus. Use it as a tea by adding ½ teaspoon savory to 1 cup boiling water. Drink only once a day.

THYME. This herb helps rid the body of mucus, strengthens the lungs to fight off infection, and acts as a shield against bacteria. Use it dried as a seasoning or make a tea by adding ¼ to ½ teaspoon thyme (it's a very strong herb, so you don't need much) to 1 cup boiling water. Steep for 5 minutes and sweeten with honey. If you have thyme oil on hand, dilute it (2 parts olive or corn oil to 1 part thyme oil) and rub on the chest to cure congestion.

CANKER SORES

That wonderful spaghetti sauce has been simmering on the burner for hours, and you can't wait for the feast to begin. Just one last taste before culinary paradise and...Zap! It got you. It stings and your eyes tear up just a bit. All your well-planned preparations have been conquered by a painful canker, squelched by stomatitis (an inflammation of the mouth), annihilated by an apthous ulcer (the medical name for a canker).

Cankers are small white sores with red edges that develop inside your mouth. They hurt like the dickens, but usually they're not serious. The most painful phase lasts about three to four days, and the sores go away in about ten days. More than 80 percent of all mouth sores are cankers, but many people confuse them with cold sores (fever blisters), which they are not.

Canker sores, unfortunately, can be repeaters, and some people are simply predisposed to getting them over and over. Most of the time the sores are not a major concern. They usually don't get infected, spread, or bleed if you don't bite them. But they're definitely a major pain.

You can find over-the-counter antiseptic creams, lozenges, and mouthwashes at your local pharmacy to help relieve canker sore pain. But you can also find some relief over the kitchen counter in some common and not so common kitchen staples.

Honey

KITCHEN CURES

CRANBERRY JUICE. Drink this juice between meals: It's both a pain reliever and canker healer.

HONEY. Mix 1 teaspoon honey with ¼ teaspoon turmeric and dab it on your canker. This one may sting a bit.

SAGE. Used most often to spice up turkey stuffing, this herb is one that can be used to calm an angry canker. Simply add 3 teaspoons sage leaves to 1 pint boiling water. Steep, covered, for 15 minutes. Rinse your mouth with the liquid several times a day. You can also rub sage leaves into a powder and apply them directly to your sore.

TEA. Moisten a regular tea bag and apply it directly to the canker. The tannic acid will help dry it out.

EDIBLE NO-NOS

Some of canker's prevailing causes are said to be spicy, sour, or acidic foods. If you develop a canker after eating pineapple or a mild sandwich that you spiced up with mustard or barbecue sauce, these could be trigger foods. Only you know what you eat before cankers pop up, so if you're plagued and can't figure out why, keep a canker sore diary. Note the foods you eat before a canker erupts and also record other facts in your life such as menstrual cycle or hormonal fluctuations, medications you took, and undue stress. You may see a pattern. In the meantime, here are a few of the foods to avoid when that canker comes calling:

- Carbonated soft drinks
- Tomatoes and tomato-based products
- Citrus fruits
- Pineapple
- Spicy foods
- Foods at a hot temperature
- Chocolate
- Foods with sharp edges: crackers, chips
- Alcoholic beverages

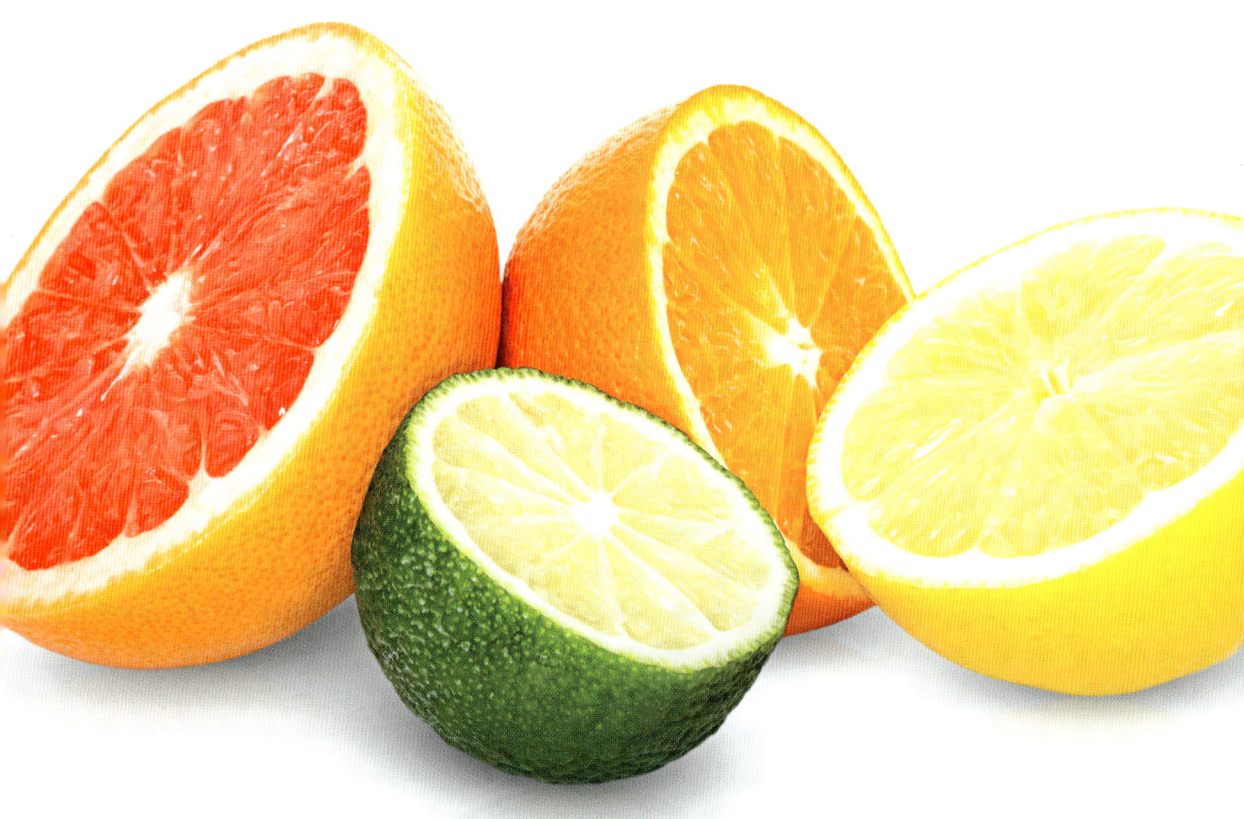

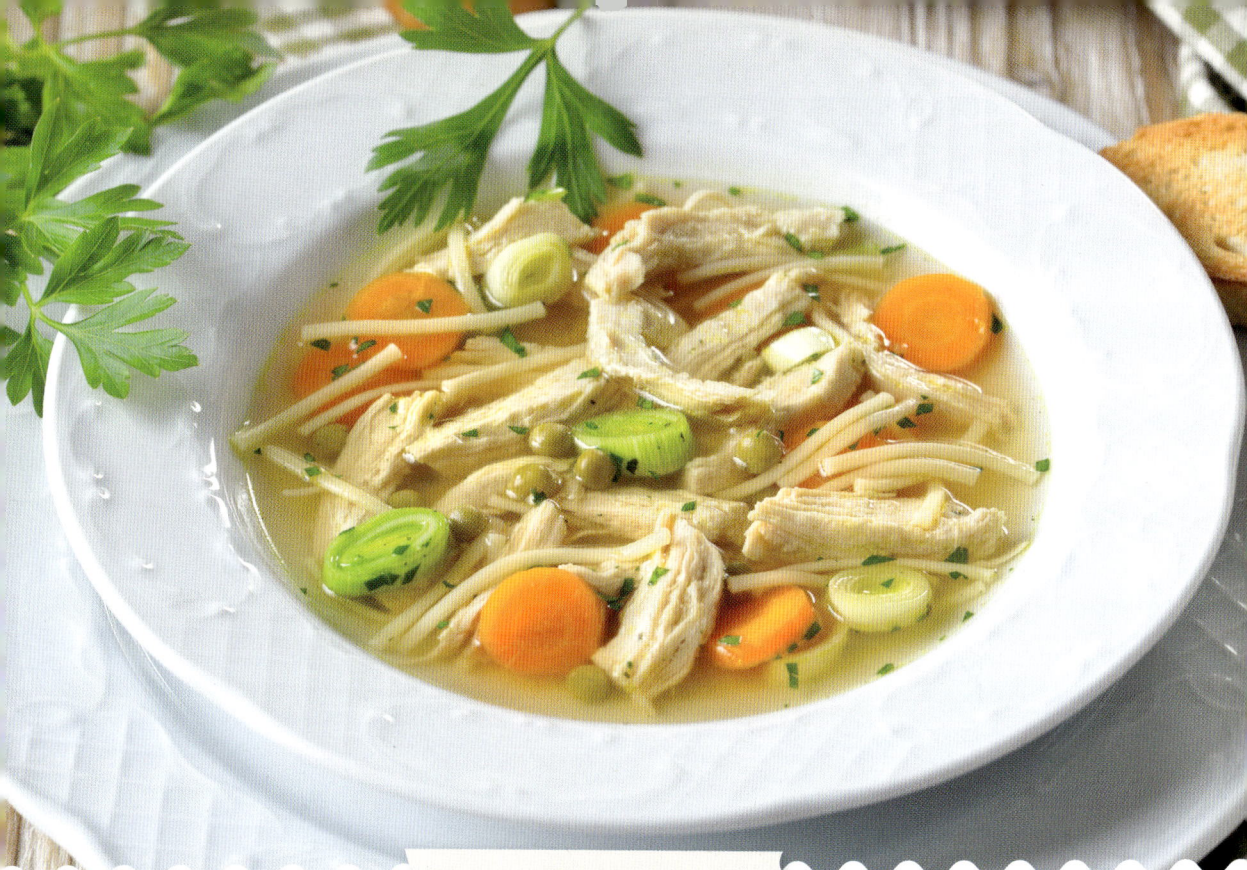

COLDS

Every year Americans will suffer through more than one billion colds. That's one billion runny noses, coughs, sneezes, aches, and sore throats. Colds make such frequent appearances that the infection has come to be known as the "common cold."

Small children are the most likely to catch a cold: Most kids will have six to ten colds a year. That's because their young immune systems combined with the germy confines of school and day-care situations make them prime targets for the virus. The upside of having so many colds as a child is that you develop immunities to some of the 200 viruses that cause colds. As a result, adults get an average of only two to four colds a year. By the time most people reach age 60, they're down to about one cold per year. Women, however, especially women between 20 and 30 years old, get more colds than men.

Thankfully, there are some things you can do to fend off the germs that cause colds, as well as techniques to ease your symptoms once you're sick.

KITCHEN CURES

CHICKEN SOUP. Science actually backs up what your mom knew all along—chicken soup does help a cold. Scientists believe it's the fumes in the soup that release the mucus in your nose and help your body better fight against its viral invaders. Chicken soup also contains cysteines, which are good at thinning mucus. And the soup provides easily absorbed nutrients.

CORN SYRUP. You can make a sugar-water gargle to ease your throat. Use 1 tablespoon syrup per 8 ounces warm water, mix together, and gargle.

HONEY. Make your own cough syrup by mixing together ¼ cup honey and ¼ cup apple cider vinegar. Pour the mixture into a jar or bottle and seal tightly. Shake well before using. Take 1 tablespoon every four hours.

PEPPERS. Hot and spicy foods are notorious for making your nose run and your eyes water. The hot stuff in peppers is called capsaicin and is pharmacologically similar to guaifenesin, an expectorant found in some over-the-counter cough syrups. This similarity leads some experts to believe that eating hot foods can clear up mucus and ease that stuffy nose.

TEA. A cup of hot tea with honey does the same trick as chicken soup; it loosens up your nasal passages and makes that stuffy nose feel better. Folk healers have known this secret for centuries. They often suggest drinking tea with spices and herbs that contain aromatic oils with antiviral properties. Try tea with elder, ginger, yarrow, mint, thyme, horsemint, bee balm, lemon balm, catnip, garlic, onions, or mustard.

YOGURT. One study found that participants who ate ¾ cup yogurt a day before and during cold season had 25 percent fewer colds. But you've got to start early and maintain your yogurt eating throughout the peak cold season.

ZINC. Studies have found that zinc may help immune cells fight a cold and may ease cold symptoms. The most effective zinc lozenges are those that contain 15 to 25 mg of zinc gluconate or zinc gluconate-glycine per lozenge. You can get the most out of your zinc lozenges if you start using them at the first sign of a cold and continue taking them for several days.

FROM THE SUPPLEMENT SHELF

Vitamin C won't prevent a cold, but research shows that it can help reduce the length and severity of symptoms. But to reap the benefits, you've got to take a lot of "C." The RDA for men and women 15 and older is 60 mg, but studies show that you'd need to take upward of 1,000 mg to 3,000 mg to get the cold-symptom-sparing rewards of vitamin C. For the short term, experts believe that wouldn't be harmful, but taking too much vitamin C for too long can cause severe diarrhea. Before loading up on vitamin C, check with your doctor.

COLD SORES

You know it's coming when you feel that notorious tingling on your lip and the accompanying itching and burning. You can't help stressing out about it; all you can think about is the pain and embarrassment those ugly cold sores cause. But there's not a darned thing you can do to stop a cold sore, also known as a fever blister, from erupting.

Many people get confused about whether they have a cold sore or a canker sore. But that confusion is easily cleared up. If the sore is on your external lip or near your mouth or nose and looks like a fluid-filled blister, chances are it's a cold sore. Caused by a virus called herpes simplex Type 1, herpes blisters are very contagious. They also love company, so where there's one there are usually many. Within a few days to a week, the blisters break, ooze, and form an ugly yellow crust that can stay around for weeks. When it finally sloughs off, though, there's nice, healthy pink skin underneath. Best of all, cold sores leave no scars.

You can't cure cold sores, and they like to keep coming back, usually to the scene of a previous visit. When a cold sore's not making itself a huge lip ache, it's snoozing in the nerves below your skin, just waiting for a reason to wake up. And what sets off its alarm clock?

- Fever
- Infection, colds, flu
- Ultraviolet radiation, such as a sunburn
- Stress
- Fatigue
- Changes in the immune system
- Trauma
- Food allergies
- Menstruation
- Dental work

Conventional medicine does have a few tricks in its little black bag, including antiviral lotions and creams. But they don't cure, just treat. So take a look in your kitchen. You might just find some useful treatments there, too.

KITCHEN CURES

LICORICE. Studies show that glycyrrhizic acid, an ingredient in licorice, stops the cold sore virus cells dead in their tracks. So try chewing a licorice whip. Just be sure it's made from real licorice, as most candy in the United States today is flavored with anise. If the ingredient list says "licorice mass," the product contains real licorice.

MILK. This remedy doesn't involve drinking. Soak a cotton ball in milk and apply it to the sore to relieve pain. Better yet, if you feel the telltale tingling before the cold sore surfaces, go straight to the cold milk. It can help speed the healing right from the beginning.

FOODS THAT FIGHT COLD SORES

There's a good amino acid, lysine, that helps block the herpes virus. So try some foods high in this cold sore warrior, such as:

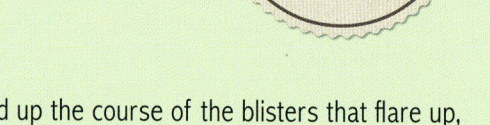

- Meats
- Milk
- Fish
- Chicken
- Eggs
- Beans & bean sprouts
- Cheese

Foods rich in bioflavonoids can help prevent or speed up the course of the blisters that flare up, too. These include:

- Onions
- Apples
- Grapes
- Tea

Foods packed with vitamin C are also valiant in their quest to rid you of your herpes foe. Eat a lot of these foods that are rich in vitamin C:

- Seedless berries (which make great smoothies)
- Peppers
- Green leafy vegetables
- Sweet potatoes and potatoes

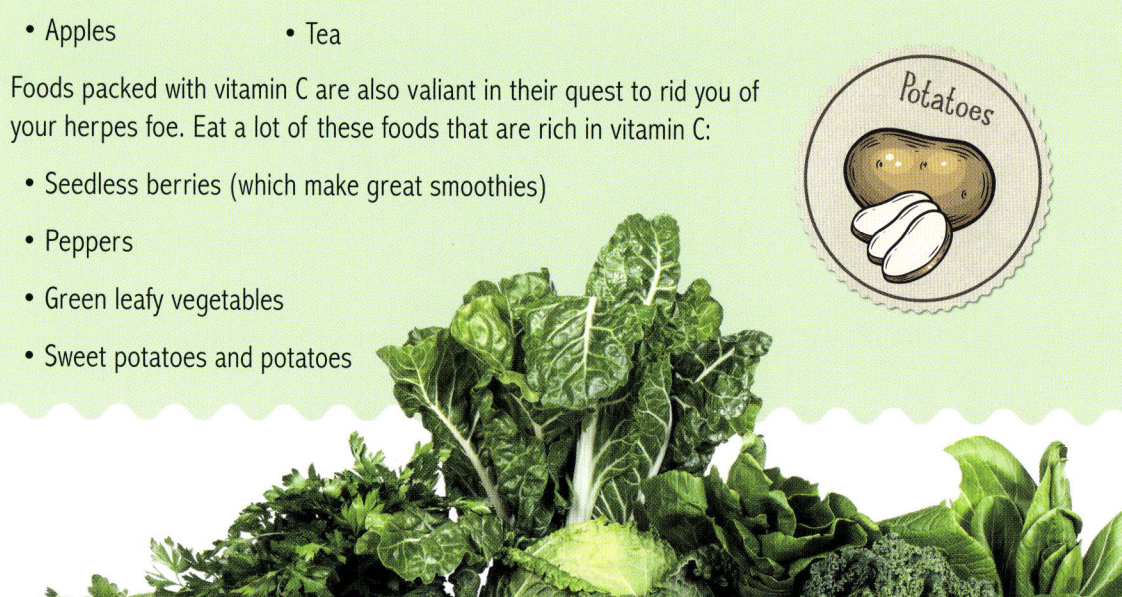

FOODS TO AVOID

During a herpes simplex episode, anything with arginine, an amino acid, is on the no-no list. Arginine causes the herpes virus to multiply. Food that contain arginine include:

- Chocolate
- Peanuts and other nuts
- Raisins
- Seeds
- Wheat and wheat products
- Oats
- Coconut
- Soy beans

Several foods that don't contain arginine can also make the episode worse. Stay away from sugar, coffee, fried foods, and alcohol. If you're prone to cold sores, stay away from tobacco, too, as it suppresses the immune system. Skip spices and spicy foods. That includes taking a pass on mustard and barbecue. Watch the acidic fruits, too, such as oranges, grapefruits, and especially pineapples.

COLIC

Bringing home a newborn baby is one of life's greatest joys. Yet it can also be one of life's greatest trials, especially if that cute little bundle of joy cries constantly. That's the number one symptom of colic: nonstop crying combined with bouts of irritability and fussiness that last a total of more than three hours a day on more than three days of the week. Colic, if it happens, typically begins at around two weeks of age and tapers off around three months. It generally is more pronounced during the evenings. Parents will be pleased to know that despite the crying, most colicky babies are healthy, well-fed infants, and the condition isn't life threatening or classified as a disease.

Unfortunately for both baby and parents, doctors don't know what causes colic, what the disorder is, or how to cure it. They don't even know if colicky babies are in pain. Fortunately for everyone involved, there are many tried-and-true ways to soothe a baby. Experiment with a few, determine what works, and stick to it.

KITCHEN CURES

BASIL. This aromatic herb contains large amounts of eugenol, which, among other things, has antispasmodic and sedative properties. Place 1 teaspoon dried basil leaves in a cup and fill it with boiling water. Cover and let stand for ten minutes. Strain and, while warm or at room temperature, give it to the infant in a bottle. A nursing mother may also drink the tea.

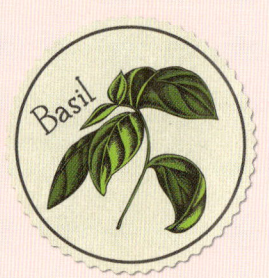

CHAMOMILE TEA. Chamomile combines antispasmodic and sedative properties and may relieve intestinal cramping and induce relaxation at the same time. In fact, chamomile contains 19 different antispasmodic constituents, as well as 5 sedative ones. To make a cup of tea: Place 1 teaspoon chamomile flowers in a cup and fill with boiling water. Cover and let stand for ten minutes. Strain and, while warm or at room temperature, give to the infant in a bottle. A nursing mother may also drink the tea, unless she is allergic to pollens. Prepackaged chamomile tea bags may be used instead of flowers.

MINT. Mint has antispasmodic properties, which may help reduce intestinal spasms in colicky infants. Place 1 teaspoon dried mint in a cup and fill with boiling water. Let stand for ten minutes. Strain well and, while warm, feed to the baby in a bottle. Nursing mothers may want to have a cup of mint tea, too. A peppermint stick soaked in water may be used as an alternative, but note that many sticks contain sugar. Never use straight peppermint oil to make tea. It's too potent for a baby.

SOY PRODUCTS. That carton of cow's milk looks innocent enough, but it can be the problem source for five to ten percent of colicky babies. Many studies have shown an improvement in colic after dairy products have been eliminated from babies' diets. The culprit seems to be the protein in cow's milk. (Don't think milk is the only villain. This protein lurks in many infant formulas containing dairy and is also found in the milk of breast-feeding mothers who consume dairy products.) Try eliminating dairy products for two weeks and switch to soy products, both for baby and for you if you're breast-feeding. If you don't notice any improvement, assume milk isn't the culprit.

WATCH WHAT YOU EAT

Many experts suggest nursing mothers look to recent dietary changes for the cause of colic. Nursing mothers should try to avoid eating the following:

- Garlic
- Onions
- Broccoli
- Cauliflower
- Cabbage
- Peanut butter
- Fish

If colic persists, avoid dairy foods and grains.

CONSTIPATION

Nothing's moving, even though you know you have to move your bowels. Everything in your body is sending you that signal. You feel bloated and uncomfortable pressure, but when you try to go, nothing happens. Or, if you do finally go, it hurts.

Constipation occurs for many different reasons. Stress, lack of exercise, certain medications, artificial sweeteners, and a diet that's lacking fiber or fluids can each be the culprit. Certain medical conditions such as an underactive thyroid, irritable bowel syndrome, diabetes, and cancer also can cause constipation. Even age is a factor. The older we get, the more prone we are to the problem.

And constipation is a problem, although it's not an illness. It's simply what happens when bowel movements are delayed, compacted, and difficult to pass.

LAXATIVES OR NO?

It's not a good idea to use laxatives as the first line of attack when you're constipated. They can become habit-forming to the point that they damage your colon. Some laxatives inhibit the effectiveness of medications you're already taking, and there are laxatives that cause inflammation to the lining of the intestine.

Conventional thinking on laxatives is that if you must take one, find one that's psyllium- or fiber-based. Psyllium is a natural fiber that's much more gentle on the system than ingredients in many of the other products available today. Or, simply look in the kitchen for relief. It's there.

KITCHEN CURES

APPLES. Eat an hour after a meal to prevent constipation. In addition, apple juice and apple cider are natural laxatives for many people. Drink up and enjoy!

BANANAS. These may relieve constipation. Try eating two ripe bananas between meals. Avoid green bananas because they're constipating.

BARLEY. It can relieve constipation as well as keep you regular, and it has cholesterol-lowering properties, too. What more could you ask of a simple grain? Buy some barley flour, flakes, and grits. Add some barley grain to vegetable soup or stew.

BLACKSTRAP MOLASSES. Take 2 tablespoons before going to bed. It has a pretty strong taste, so you may want to add it to milk, fruit juice, or for an extra-powerful laxative punch, prune juice.

GARLIC. In the raw, it has a laxative effect for many. Eat it mixed with onion, raw or cooked, and with milk or yogurt for best results.

HONEY. This is a very mild laxative. Try taking 1 tablespoon three times a day, either by itself or mixed into warm water. If it doesn't work on its own, you may have to pep it up by mixing it half and half with blackstrap molasses.

OIL. Safflower, soybean, or other vegetable oil can be just the cure you need, as they have a lubricating action in the intestines. Take 2 to 3 tablespoons a day until the problem is gone. If you don't like taking it straight, mix the oil with herbs and lemon juice or vinegar to use as salad dressing. The combination of the oil and the fiber from the salad ought to fix you right up.

PRUNES. Yep, they work! And here's a great-tasting way to cure constipation. Cover several prunes with boiling water. If you wish to sweeten the prunes, stir 1 or 2 teaspoons honey into the boiling water before you pour it over the fruit. Let the prunes stand in the water overnight, and eat them the next day. Drink the prune juice, too. This works with figs, as well.

RAISINS. Eat a handful daily, an hour after a meal.

RHUBARB. This is a natural laxative. Cook it and eat it sweetened with honey or bake it in a pie. Or, create a drink with cooked, pureed rhubarb, apple juice, and honey.

SESAME SEED. These provide roughage and bulk, and they soften the contents of the intestines, which makes elimination easier. Eat no more than ½ ounce daily, and drink lots of water as you take the seeds. You may also sprinkle them on salads and other foods, but again, no more than ½ ounce. Sesame is also available in a butter or paste and in Middle Eastern dips, such as tahini.

VINEGAR. Mix 1 teaspoon apple cider vinegar and 1 teaspoon honey in a glass of water and drink.

WALNUTS. Fresh from the shell, they may be just the laxative you need.

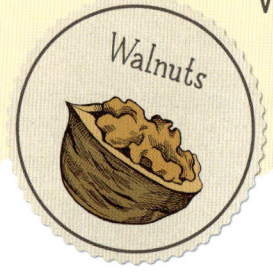

COUGH

A cough is produced when viruses, bacteria, dust, pollen, or other foreign substances irritate respiratory passages in the throat and lungs. The cough reflex is the body's effort to rid the passageways of such intruders, and it spares no power in the expulsion. A cough reflex can expel a foreign substance at velocities as high as 100 miles per hour.

Determine what kind of cough you have and search out cures specific to that type. Some remedies aim to moisten dry throats, while others are expectorants, helping you cough up and get rid of mucus and irritants. Most of these kitchen cures aim to battle both coughs unless otherwise noted.

KITCHEN CURES

CHICKEN SOUP. Take some advice from your grandma: Sip a bowl of chicken soup. It doesn't matter if it's homemade or canned. Chicken soup is calming for coughs associated with colds. While scientists can't put a finger on why this comfort food benefits the cold sufferer, they do believe chicken soup contains anti-inflammatory properties that help prevent a cold's miserable side effects, one being the cough. Plus, chicken soup contains cysteine, which thins phlegm. The broth, chock-full of electrolytes, keeps you hydrated, and the steam helps soothe irritated mucous membranes and air passageways. Last, but not least, it tastes yummy.

GARLIC. Eating garlic won't have you winning any kissing contests, but who wants to kiss you when you sound like a seal? Since kissing isn't on your agenda, you can indulge in one of nature's best cures for coughs: garlic. It's full of antibiotic and antiviral properties, plus garlic is also an expectorant, so it helps you cough up stubborn bacteria and/or mucus that are languishing in your lungs.

A cup of garlic broth may do the trick for your cough, too, and it is easy to prepare. Smash 1 to 3 cloves garlic (depending on how strong you like your garlic), add 2 quarts water, and boil on low heat for one hour. Strain and sip slowly.

You can also chop up some garlic cloves and toss them into that pot of chicken soup.

GINGER. Ginger, which has antiviral properties, shares the limelight with licorice in the cough remedy on the following page.

HONEY. Honey has long been used in traditional Chinese medicine for coughs because it's a natural expectorant, promoting the flow of mucus. This is the simple recipe: Mix 1 tablespoon honey into 1 cup hot water and enjoy. Now how sweet is that? Squeeze some lemon juice in if you want a little tartness. Before bedtime, adults may add 1 tablespoon brandy or whiskey to aid in sleep.

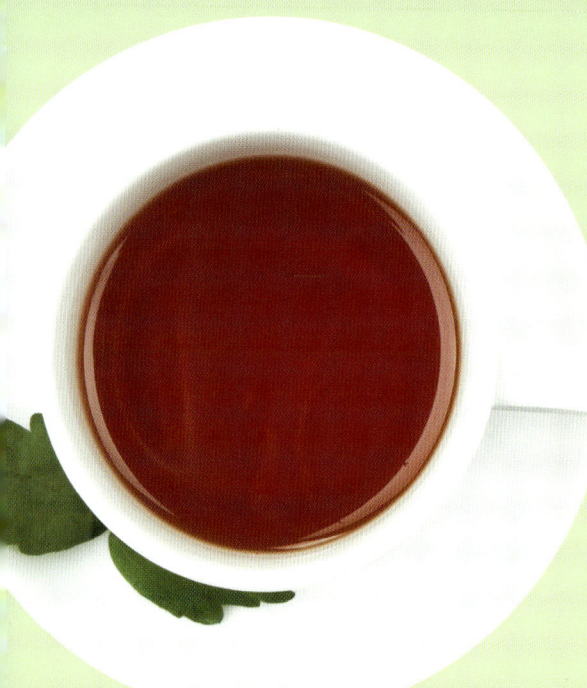

GINGER-LICORICE (ANISE) TEA:
Combine 2 teaspoons freshly chopped gingerroot, 2 teaspoons aniseed, and if available, 1 teaspoon dried licorice root in 2 cups boiling water. Cover and steep for ten minutes. Strain and sweeten with 1 or 2 teaspoons honey. Drink ½ cup every one to two hours, but no more than 3 cups a day.

LICORICE. If you love licorice, you're in for a treat with this remedy. Many folk remedies use licorice root to treat coughs and bronchial problems. It serves not only as a flavoring agent but also as a demulcent (a substance that soothes inflamed or irritated throats) and an expectorant. Real licorice or candy that's actually made with real licorice (look for licorice mass on the label) works best. Reach into your candy jar and slice up 1 ounce licorice sticks. Add 1 quart boiling water and steep for 24 hours. Drink throughout the day, adding a teaspoon of honey for sweetness.

MUSTARD SEED. An irritating but useful spice for wet coughs, mustard seed has sulfur-containing compounds that stimulate the flow of mucus. To get the full effect of the expectorant compounds, the mustard seeds must be broken and allowed to sit in water for 15 minutes. Crush 1 teaspoon mustard seeds or grind them in a coffee grinder. Place the seeds in a cup of warm water. Steep for 15 minutes. This concoction might be a little hard to swallow, so take it in ¼-cup doses throughout the day.

Mustard Seed

PEPPER. Pepper is a bit of an irritant (try sniffling some), but this characteristic is a plus for those suffering from coughs accompanied by thick mucus. The irritating property of pepper stimulates circulation and the flow of mucus in the airways and sinuses. Place 1 teaspoon black pepper into a cup and sweeten things up with the addition of 1 tablespoon honey. Fill with boiling water, steep for 10 to 15 minutes, stir, and sip.

DEHYDRATION

Every cell in your body needs water in order to function properly. In fact, an adult's body weight is 60 percent water while an infant's is up to 80 percent water. Other than oxygen, there's nothing that your body needs more than water. Water is so important because it has many critical functions in the body.

Because water has so many life-sustaining functions, dehydration isn't just a matter of being a little thirsty. The effects depend on the degree of dehydration, but a water shortage causes your kidneys to conserve water, which in turn can affect other body systems. You'll urinate less and can become constipated. As you become increasingly more dehydrated, these symptoms will develop:

- Diminished muscular endurance
- Dizziness
- Lack of energy
- Decreased concentration
- Drowsiness
- Irritability
- Headache
- Tachycardia (galloping heart rate)
- Increased body temperature
- Collapse
- Permanent organ damage or death

HOW MUCH IS ENOUGH?

Obviously, you don't want to develop the problems listed above, so you have to ask: How much water do I need each day? Under normal conditions, the standard of 64 ounces a day is sufficient. That amount includes water from sources other than the tap. A good way to tell if you're adequately hydrated is by observing the color of your urine. If it's dark yellow or amber, that's a sign that it's concentrated, meaning there's not enough water in the wastes that are being eliminated. If it's light, the color of lemon juice, that's normal. Urine will usually be darker in the morning, and lighten through the day as you drink and get fluid from foods.

KITCHEN CURES

BANANAS. They have great water content and are especially good for restoring potassium that has vanished with dehydration.

BLAND FOODS. If you've experienced dehydration, stick to foods that are easily digested for the next 24 hours because stomach cramps are a symptom and can recur. Try soda crackers, rice, bananas, potatoes, and flavored gelatins. Gelatins are especially good since they are primarily made of water.

BOTTLED WATER. Freeze some in the bottom of an empty bottle, then top if off with cold water when you're ready to go. You'll have cold water ready to drink for hours. If you know you'll need more than one bottle of cold water, grab another full bottle, drain about an inch from the top and freeze the whole thing. By the time the first bottle is empty, you'll have plenty of cold water in the second.

DECAFFEINATED TEA. Just another tasty way to get fluids in your body. Don't drink caffeinated tea, however, as caffeine is a mild diuretic.

FRUIT JUICE. It's liquid and has essential vitamins and minerals that need to be replenished.

ICE. Suck on it, or rub it on your body when you're overheated. This will help cool you down and prevent excess evaporation, which may lead to dehydration.

LIME JUICE. Add 1 teaspoon lime juice, a pinch of salt, and 1 teaspoon sugar to a pint of water. Sip the beverage throughout the day to cure mild dehydration.

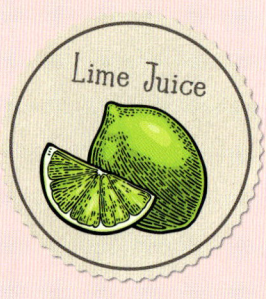

RAISINS. They're packed with potassium, a body salt lost during dehydration.

POPSICLE. A great way to restore water to your body. It's an easy way to get fluids into kids, too.

SALT. If you're experiencing symptoms of mild dehydration or heat injury, or you're just plain sweating a lot, make sure you replace your salt. Don't just chug salt straight from the box, however. Try eating pretzels, salted crackers, or salty nuts.

SPORTS DRINKS. Not only will they add water back into your system, they'll restore potassium and other essential electrolytes (a salt substance, such as potassium, sodium, and chlorine found in blood, tissue fluids, and cells that carry electrical impulses). For children, these adult drinks may be too harsh, so talk to your pharmacist about pediatric rehydration drinks now on the market.

WATERY FRUITS. Bananas are the number one fruit for rehydration, but watery fruits are a delicious and nutritious way to restore fluids. Try cantaloupe, watermelon, and strawberries. Watery vegetables such as cucumbers are good, too.

YOGURT. Or, cottage cheese. These have both sodium and potassium for replacing electrolytes.

MORE DO'S & DON'TS

- Don't cut back on your water intake if you're retaining fluids. Water retention that's caused by salt needs to be addressed by increasing water consumption to flush salt from the body.

- Drink even when you're not thirsty. You're losing body fluids every second of the day, and they must be replaced.

- Don't depend on sport drinks or soft drinks for all your fluid requirements. They can come with side effects and calories. Plain old water is the best choice.

DIABETES

Diabetes is a disease that reduces, or stops, the body's ability to produce or respond to insulin, a hormone produced in the pancreas. Insulin's role is to open the door for glucose, a form of sugar, to enter the body's cells so that it can be used for energy. When the body has a problem metabolizing glucose, it builds up in the blood, and the body's cells starve.

There are two major types of diabetes:

Type 1. The body produces no insulin at all, and daily insulin shots are required. This disease used to be called juvenile diabetes because there is a higher rate of diagnosis among children ages 10 to 14. It is also referred to as insulin-dependent diabetes because injections of insulin are required to control blood glucose. The cause isn't known, but Type 1 tends to run in families. A much smaller number of people with diabetes have Type 1—only five percent.

Type 2. This is the most common form of diabetes, and it occurs when the body is insulin resistant. That could be either because the body fails to make enough insulin or because it doesn't properly use the insulin it does produce. The cause is often poor dietary habits, sedentary lifestyle, and obesity. Those with Type 2 may or may not need oral medication or insulin, depending on how their body responds to changes in diet and exercise.

Here's the risk list for diabetes. Do any of these describe you?

- Over age 45
- Family history of diabetes
- Overweight
- Don't exercise regularly
- Low HDL cholesterol or high triglycerides
- Member of an at-risk ethnic group

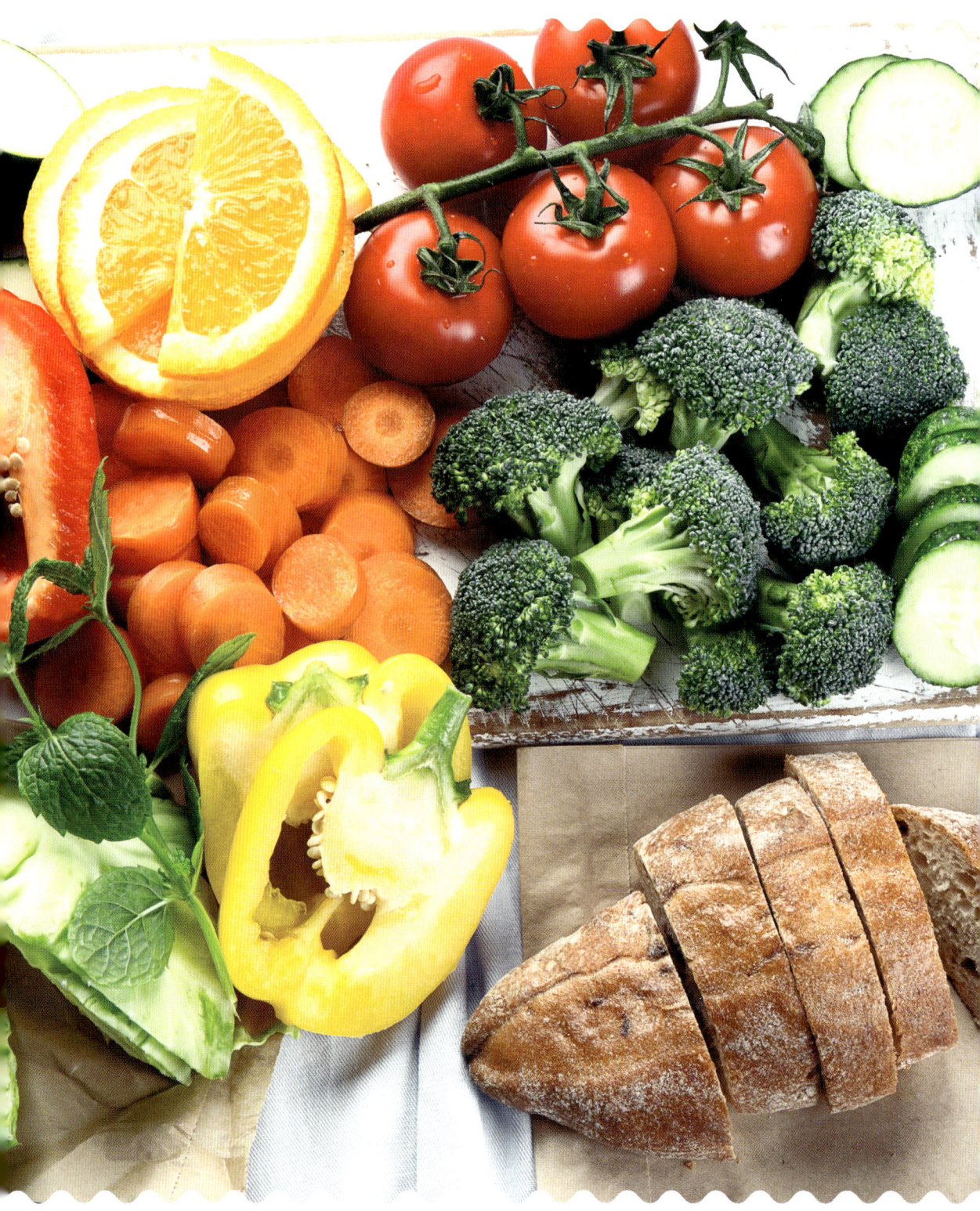

TREATMENT

While there is no easy cure for diabetes, it can be controlled and even reversed. And control is essential because diabetes can lead to heart disease, stroke, kidney disease and failure, blindness, and amputation if not treated. This profile will not address diabetic medical treatment, including prescribed diabetic diets. Those specifics must be left up to your physician and dietitian. But this profile will cover the go-alongs; things from your kitchen that can make the diabetic experience easier. Note, however, that nothing contained in this profile is intended to stop or replace your prescribed diabetic care!

Diabetes is a complex disease, affecting many parts of the body. Some of the problems of the disease can be relieved with simple things right from the kitchen, though. And for a person with diabetes, a little relief never hurts.

KITCHEN CURES

ASPARAGUS. This vegetable is a mild diuretic that's said to be beneficial in the control of diabetes. Eat it steamed and drizzled with olive oil and lemon juice.

BEANS. They've been known to reduce blood sugar in some people. Kidney beans are the best, fresh in the pod. Boil 2 ounces of sliced pods in 4 quarts of water. Simmer four hours. Strain and cool the liquid for eight hours. Strain again. Drink 1 glassful every two hours. In the absence of kidney bean pods, fresh green beans will work, too. Beans eaten with a meal have been known to lessen the rise in blood sugar that comes after the meal.

GARLIC. Eating a combination of garlic, parsley, and watercress may shave a few points off the blood sugar. Try combining these herbs in a vegetable stir-fry or salad.

LEMON. A tasty substitute for salt. It's great squeezed into a diet cola, too. It cuts the aftertaste.

OLIVE OIL. Studies indicate this may reduce blood sugar levels. Use it in salad dressing or wherever cooking oils are indicated. For an inexpensive and easy no-stick olive oil spray-on coating, buy an oil mister in any department store kitchen supply area and use it to spray your pans before cooking.

PARSLEY. Steep into a tea and drink. This may act as a diuretic as well as lower blood sugar.

PEANUT BUTTER. After you've experienced an episode of low blood sugar and corrected it, follow up with a protein and carbohydrate snack. Peanut butter on a couple of crackers supplies both, and it's easy to fix when you may still feel a little jittery. Just avoid brands that contain added sugar, glucose, or jelly.

SALT SHAKER. Set it aside, put it back in the cupboard, hide it. High blood pressure is a side effect of diabetes, and that salt's a no-no. So don't cook with it, and don't make it handy to grab when you eat a meal or snack. If it's out of sight, or inconvenient to get, you might just skip it. Instead, reach for a nice herb or spice blend that's sodium free. Make one yourself with your favorite spices or buy one at the store.

SUGAR. Yes, even people with diabetes need it occasionally, when their blood sugar goes too low. A spoonful of straight sugar will work, as will a piece of hard candy. Just be sure it's not sugarless.

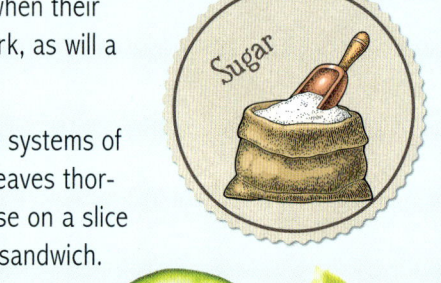

WATERCRESS. This is said to strengthen the natural defense systems of people who have diabetes. It's also a mild diuretic. Wash the leaves thoroughly, and add them to a salad. Or smear a little cream cheese on a slice of bread, then top with watercress for a delicious open-faced sandwich.

MORE DO'S AND DON'TS

- Use a fork to apply salad dressing and sauces to limit your intake of sugar, as well as fat and cholesterol. Instead of dumping the dressing or sauce all over your food, have it served "on the side" and dip your fork into it, then pick up your food. You'll get the flavor without all the extra goop.

- Use a notebook to keep track of glucose readings, medication schedules, and symptoms.

- Monitor your glucose levels regularly via finger sticks. That's the only way you can accurately gauge how you're doing. Record the results for your doctor and dietician.

- Maintain a regular eating schedule. Your body needs it.

- Eat foods with a low glycemic index, as they release sugar slowly into the bloodstream.

- If your blood sugar level drops to the point that you need a quick pick-me-up, candy's fine, but skip the chocolate. Its high fat content slows the absorption of sugar, so it doesn't work quickly enough.

- As fruits are dehydrated, the sugar in them becomes concentrated. Limit your intake of dried fruit to two or three times a week or less.

DIARRHEA

Diarrhea is probably one of the most unpleasant problems that plagues us, and it's a common malady. Americans usually suffer from diarrhea a couple times a year. For most adults, diarrhea isn't serious. And it does give you a chance to ponder some redecorating ideas for the bathroom.

There are essentially two types of diarrhea: acute and chronic. Thankfully, the vast majority of diarrhea is acute, or short term. This type of diarrhea keeps you on the toilet for a couple of days but doesn't stick around long. Acute diarrhea is also known as non-inflammatory diarrhea. Its symptoms are what most people associate with the condition: watery, frequent stools accompanied by stomach cramps, gas, and nausea.

Acute diarrhea usually has a bacterial or viral culprit. Gastroenteritis, mistakenly called the "stomach flu," is one of the most common infections that cause diarrhea. Gastroenteritis can be caused by many different viruses. Eating or drinking foods contaminated with bacteria can also cause diarrhea. Other causes of acute diarrhea are lactose intolerance, sweeteners such as sorbitol, over-the-counter antacids that contain magnesium, too much vitamin C, and some antibiotics.

If you have chronic, or long-term, diarrhea that comes on suddenly and stays for weeks, you may have a more serious condition such as irritable bowel syndrome or a severe food allergy.

DEHYDRATION DANGERS

With any kind of diarrhea you lose a lot of fluids. One of the quickest ways you can end up going from the bathroom to the emergency room is to take a pass on liquids while you're sick. Fluids not only keep things running smoothly in your body, they also keep electrolyte levels balanced. Electrolytes are sodium, potassium, and chloride salts that your body needs for proper organ function. An electrolyte imbalance can cause your heart to beat irregularly, causing life-threatening problems. Though drinking or eating anything while you're running back and forth to the bathroom might sound grotesque, it will help make you more comfortable and get you back on your feet more quickly.

Though experts don't see eye to eye on what fluids are best during a bout with diarrhea, they do agree that getting two to three quarts of fluid a day is a good idea. When you drink, it's easier on the tummy if you sip instead of gulp (who has the energy for gulping?) and if you drink cool, not cold or hot, fluids. Here are some tried-and-true fluids that should get you through the rough days.

- Decaffeinated tea with a little sugar
- Sports drinks
- Commercially available electrolyte replacement drinks for children
- Bouillon
- Chicken broth

Though it may not sound logical to put diarrhea and food in the same sentence, if you don't put something in your body while you're enduring tummy troubles, you might end up getting sicker. There are loads of good things from the kitchen that will ease your grumbling stomach.

KITCHEN CURES

BANANA. Long known as a soother for tummy trouble, this potassium-rich fruit can restore nutrients and is easy to digest.

BLUEBERRIES. Blueberry root is a long-time folk remedy for diarrhea. In Sweden, doctors prescribe a soup made with dried blueberries for tummy problems. Blueberries are rich in anthocyanosides, which have antioxidant and antibacterial properties, as well as tannins, which combat diarrhea.

CHAMOMILE TEA. Chamomile is good for treating intestinal inflammation, and it has antispasmodic properties as well. You can brew yourself a cup of chamomile tea from packaged tea bags, or you can buy chamomile flowers and steep 1 teaspoon of them and 1 teaspoon of peppermint leaves in a cup of boiling water for fifteen minutes. Drink 3 cups a day.

COOKED CEREALS. Starchy foods, such as precooked rice or tapioca cereals, can help ease your tummy. Prepare the cereal according to the directions on the box, making it as thick as you can stomach it. Just avoid adding too much sugar or salt, as these can aggravate diarrhea. It's probably a good idea to avoid oatmeal since it's high in fiber and your intestines can't tolerate the added bulk during a bout with diarrhea.

FENUGREEK SEEDS. Science has given the nod to this folk remedy. But this one is for adults only. Mix ½ teaspoon fenugreek seeds with water and drink up.

ORANGE PEEL. Orange peel tea is a folk remedy that is believed to aid in digestion. Place a chopped orange peel (preferably from an organic orange, as peels otherwise may contain pesticides and dyes) into a pot and cover with 1 pint boiling water. Let it stand until the water is cooled. You can sweeten it with sugar or honey.

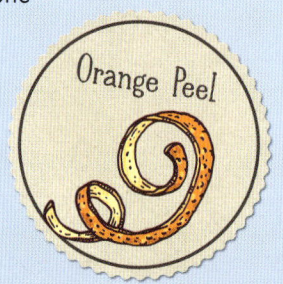

POTATOES. This is another starchy food that can help restore nutrients and comfort your stomach. But eating french fries won't help. Fried foods tend to aggravate an aching tummy. Other root vegetables such as carrots (cooked, of course) are also easy on an upset stomach, and they are loaded with nutrients.

RICE. Cooked white rice is another starchy food that can be handled by someone recovering from diarrhea.

SUGAR. To make your own fluid replacement, mix 4 teaspoons sugar and ½ teaspoon salt with 1 quart water. Mixing electrolytes (such as salt) with a form of glucose (sugar) helps the body to better absorb the nutrients.

YOGURT. Look for yogurt with live cultures. These "cultures" are friendly bacteria that can go in and line your intestines, providing you protection from the bad guys. If you've already got diarrhea, yogurt can help produce lactic acid in your intestines, which can kill off the nasty bacteria and get you feeling better, faster.

DRY MOUTH

Dry mouth, also known as xerostomia, is a condition in which saliva production shuts down. When working at full capacity, saliva has many duties. This versatile fluid helps us talk, chew, and spit. It acts as a natural cavity fighter by washing away food particles and plaque, and it lubricates food, works to buffer acids, and re-mineralizes those pearly whites. Saliva is vital in maintaining a healthy mouth, so when production decreases or stops, there is more than a dry mouth to pout about. Teeth and gums become more prone to decay and infection, and your taste buds might suffer in their taste-testing abilities.

WHAT CAUSES DRY MOUTH?

Dry mouth is caused by several factors, most commonly by the use of medications. Look on almost any label of nonprescription and prescription drugs, and you'll find that dry mouth is typically listed as a possible side effect. Some of the worst offenders are those drugs designed to dry out your mucous membranes, such as antihistamines and many allergy medications. Other drugs contributing to dryness are those used to treat high blood pressure, depression, and heart disease.

Other causes of xerostomia are radiation therapy, menopause, surgical removal of the salivary glands, and cigarette smoking.

KITCHEN CURES

ANISEED. Munching on aniseed can help combat the bad breath that accompanies dry mouth. In fact, many Indian restaurants have a bowl of anise and fennel available to remove pungent food odors from your breath. Mix a few teaspoons of these seeds, place in a covered bowl, and keep on the table.

CAYENNE PEPPER. A dry mouth often inhibits taste buds from distinguishing between sour, sweet, salty, and bitter flavors. A mouthwatering method to stimulate saliva production and bolster those buds is to sprinkle red pepper (cayenne) on your food or mix it into your favorite juice (tomato juice seems most compatible). Better yet, prepare an entire meal around red pepper, which acts as nature's wake-up call, stimulating salivary glands, sweat glands, and tear ducts. Go south of the border with some spicy salsas or make that all-American favorite, chili, and start drooling!

CELERY. If you need an excuse to snack, here it is! Munching on such waterlogged snacks as celery sticks helps stimulate the saliva glands and adds moisture to your mouth. Should your sweet tooth strike, suck on sugarless candies. Definitely stay away from sugar-filled treats since they promote decay in an already vulnerable mouth.

FENNEL. Munching on fennel seeds mixed with aniseed can help combat bad breath that accompanies dry mouth. In addition, fennel seed can be combined with other herbs to make a mouthwash.

LIQUIDS. If the salivary glands are down for the count, you'll need all the reinforcements you can muster to help get food down. Try to complement each dish with sauce, gravy, broth, butter, or yogurt. Food will be easier to swallow. Another option is to stick to soft, liquidy foods, such as stews, soups, and noodle dishes.

PARSLEY. A dry mouth is not only uncomfortable, but it often brings out bad breath. This double whammy can ruin just about any social situation. Luckily, battling bad breath is easy. See that parsley on your plate? The restaurant may put it there for decoration, but it can serve a more useful purpose. This herb is a natural breath sweetener, and it provides ample amounts of vitamins A and C, calcium, and iron. So, chew on some.

ROSEMARY. Store-bought mouthwash overflows with germ-killing alcohol, which is also a drying agent. Read labels and don't purchase any that contain alcohol. Better yet, reach into your spice rack and pull out rosemary, mint, and aniseed to make a refreshing herbal mouthwash. The rosemary helps fight germs, while the mint and aniseed freshen breath.

Combine 1 teaspoon dried rosemary, 1 teaspoon dried mint, and 1 teaspoon aniseed with 2½ cups boiling water. Cover and steep for 15 to 20 minutes. Strain and refrigerate. Use as a gargle.

WATER. Tap or bottled, whatever way you drink water is fine...just drink plenty of it. To keep your system well lubricated, it's recommended you down eight, 8-ounce glasses each day. Cut back on other refreshments such as coffee, sugary sodas, and alcohol, all of which can exacerbate dry mouth. Make sure to accompany every meal with a glass of water.

DRINKS TO AVOID

Cut down on coffee and alcohol consumption. Both are diuretics and can leave your mouth feeling as dry as the Sahara.

FEVER

Fever is a good thing. It's your body's attempt to kill off invading bacteria and other nasty organisms that can't survive the heat. The hypothalamus, which is the body's thermostat, senses the assault on the body and turns up the heat much the way you turn up the thermostat when you feel cold. It's a simple defense mechanism, and the sweat that comes with a fever is merely a way to cool the body down.

It used to be standard medical practice to knock that fever out as quickly as possible. Not so anymore. The value of fever is recognized, and since a fever will usually subside when the infection that's causing it runs its course, modern thinking is to ride out that fever, especially if it stays under 102°F in adults. However, if a fever is making you uncomfortable or interfering with your ability to eat, drink, or sleep, treat it. Your body needs adequate nutrition, hydration, and rest to fight the underlying cause of the fever.

Fever is a symptom, not an illness, and so there's no specific cure. But there are some fever-relievers in the kitchen that may make you feel better for the duration. Be aware that the most significant side effect of fever is dehydration.

KITCHEN CURES

APPLE WATER. It tastes good, relieves the miseries of fever, and keeps the body hydrated. To make it, peel, skin, core, and slice 3 sweet apples. Put them in a pan with 3¾ cups water. Bring to a boil, then simmer until the apples are barely mushy. Remove, strain without pressing apple puree into the liquid, and add 2 tablespoons honey. Drink and enjoy.

BASIL. Mix 1 teaspoon basil with ¼ teaspoon black pepper. Steep in 1 cup hot water to make a tea. Add 1 teaspoon honey. Drink two to three times a day.

BLACKBERRY VINEGAR. This is a great fever elixir, but it takes several days to prepare. Pour cider vinegar over a pound or two of blackberries, then cover the container and store it in a cool, dark place for three days. Strain for a day, since it takes time for all the liquid to drain from the berries, and collect the liquid in another container. Then add 2 cups sugar to each 2½ cups juice. Bring to a boil, then simmer for 5 minutes while you skim the scum off the top. Cool and store in an airtight jar in a cool place. Mix 1 teaspoonful with water to quench the thirst caused by a fever.

CREAM OF TARTAR. Try this fever tea. Combine 1½ teaspoons cream of tartar, ½ teaspoon lemon juice, 2½ cups warm water, and ½ teaspoon honey. Drink 4 to 6 ounces at a time.

GINGER. This can help break a high fever. Grate 2 tablespoons fresh ginger and add to 2 cups boiling water. Steep 30 minutes. Add a little honey to sweeten, and drink a cup of the warm beverage every two to three hours.

FRUIT JUICE. It will replace the fluids lost through sweating. Lemonade is a good choice, too.

LETTUCE. Pour a pint of boiling water over an entire head of lettuce and let it steep, covered, for 15 minutes. Strain, sweeten the liquid to taste, and drink. In addition to keeping you hydrated, this lettuce infusion may help you sleep better.

OREGANO. A tea made from a mixture of some spice rack staples can help reduce fever. Steep 1 teaspoon each of oregano and marjoram in a pint of boiling water for 30 minutes. Strain, and drink warm a couple times a day. Refrigerate unused portion until needed, then gently warm.

PINEAPPLE. Fresh is best. It's one of nature's anti-inflammatory agents that can fight fever. Pineapple is also packed with juice that can prevent dehydration.

POPSICLE. These can reduce the risk of dehydration. Fruit juice bars are good, too. This can be an especially handy way to keep fluids in small children.

RAISINS. Drink a little of this several times a day to keep yourself hydrated during a fever. Put ¾ cup chopped raisins in 7½ cups water. Bring to a boil, then simmer until the water has been reduced by one-third.

SAGE. Mix 2 teaspoons dried sage with 1 teaspoon dried peppermint. Pour 1 cup boiling water over these and steep 15 minutes. Strain and sweeten with honey. Drink 2 to 3 cups per day, re-warmed. Add a little honey to sweeten the taste.

WATER. Drink lots of it to prevent dehydration. Sponging the body with lukewarm water can relieve fever symptoms, but it's recommended that you use fever-reducing medication first to reduce the possibility of chills and shivering. Do not use cold water or ice on the body.

MORE DO'S & DON'TS

- Skip the alcohol and caffeine. They're diuretics, and you don't need to lose more fluid.
- If you don't feel like eating, don't, even though your mother told you to feed that fever and starve that cold. Just make sure you get sufficient fluids. Do reintroduce yourself to foods gradually, though, if you haven't been eating very much.

FLATULENCE

Bodily gas originates in the stomach and travels down to the intestines (unless it comes back up as a belch). Its construction is pretty simple: carbon dioxide, hydrogen, nitrogen, and methane. Those gases make up about 99 percent of the gas we pass. The other 1 percent is divided among up to 250 different gases, all of which occur naturally when carbohydrates are broken down. If you swallow air, you add oxygen to the mix.

Gas normally has no odor, but some foods simply hang around in the intestines too long and begin to ferment. Fermentation causes the offensive odor that sometimes occurs. And the more food that's fermenting, the more volume of gas building up for its grand exit.

Gas is a side effect or symptom, not an illness in itself. And it's a symptom that can be treated several different ways with things you find in the kitchen.

KITCHEN CURES

CARAWAY CRACKERS. Caraway seeds and their oils are carminatives (they get rid of gas), but who wants to eat just the seeds? Caraway seed crackers and breads with caraway seeds are a tasty way to make your system gas-unfriendly.

CARDAMOM SEEDS. These speed digestion. Add them to sautéed vegetables or to rice or lentils before cooking. You can also chew whole pods or steep pods in boiling water for several minutes to make a tea.

CLOVES. They pep up digestion and eliminate gas. Add 2 to 3 whole cloves to rice before cooking. Sprinkle on apples and pears when baking. Or steep 2 to 3 whole cloves in a cup of boiling water for ten minutes, sweeten to taste, and drink.

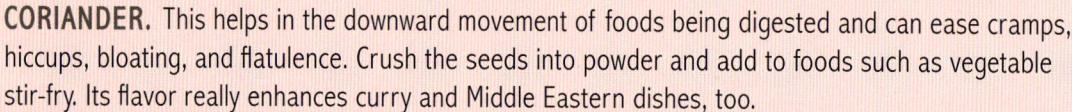

CITRUS FRUITS. Vitamin C in tablet form may cause gas, especially amounts in excess of 500 milligrams. So, reduce the dosage and replace the C with these high-in-C fruits. Also try the following vegetables, which are high in vitamin C: potatoes, sweet peppers.

CORIANDER. This helps in the downward movement of foods being digested and can ease cramps, hiccups, bloating, and flatulence. Crush the seeds into powder and add to foods such as vegetable stir-fry. Its flavor really enhances curry and Middle Eastern dishes, too.

FENNEL SEEDS. It's an acquired taste, but it may be one well worth acquiring if you're plagued by gas. Fennel's digestive powers are so good that in India fennel is customarily eaten after a meal to help digestion and freshen the breath. For gas, drink it as a tea by steeping ½ teaspoon seeds in 1 cup boiling water for ten minutes. Or, sprinkle them over those gassy vegetables during cooking or add to stir-fries. If you've acquired the taste, fennel also works well cooked into figs, apples, pears, and plums.

GINGER. Combine 1 teaspoon fresh grated ginger with 1 teaspoon lime juice. Take after eating.

LEMON. Stir 1 teaspoon lemon juice and ½ teaspoon baking soda into 1 cup cool water. Skip the ice water; it can start digestive spasms that cause gas. Drink after meals.

PUMPKIN. It soothes the tummy, and best of all, it cuts down on flatulence. Try some baked, steamed, or broiled. Or, make yourself a simple pumpkin soup.

ROSEMARY. If you're eating a gassy food, sprinkle on a little rosemary to cut down the effect. You can do the same with sage and thyme, too.

TEA HERBS. Steep and drink a tea made from any of these: aniseed, basil leaves, chamomile, cloves, cinnamon, ginger, peppermint, sage. Steep about ½ teaspoon in 1 cup boiling water, then add honey or lemon to taste. Drink one to three times each day.

TURMERIC. This may stop a gas problem altogether. Turmeric is one of the many flavorful and curative spices found in curry powder. You can add turmeric itself to rice or season a bland dish with curry powder, which contains turmeric. However you use it, it helps alleviate gas.

YOGURT WITH ACIDOPHILUS. It alleviates digestive woes, including gas. But the yogurt must have live acidophilus, a bacteria that helps with digestion.

MORE DO'S & DON'TS

- Try cutting back some on fiber, especially from legumes. Fiber is good for you, but increasing fiber intake too quickly can cause gas.

- Reduce the amount of fermented foods you eat, such as cheese, soy sauce, and alcohol.

- Cut back on carbonated beverages.

- Don't stuff yourself when you eat. The more food in the gut, the more gas buildup. And eat more slowly—you'll swallow less air.

- Don't sip drinks through a straw. You'll suck in air, which causes gas.

FLATULOGENIC FOODS

If you're plagued by gas, here are some foods that are definitely on the top of the flatus-maker list:

- Beer
- Bran
- Broccoli
- Brussels sprouts
- Cabbage
- Carbonated drinks
- Cauliflower
- Corn
- Legumes (beans, lentils, dried peas)
- Milk
- Onions
- Rutabaga

THE BENEFIT OF BEANS

Thinking about giving beans the boot? Don't do it! Beans are loaded with cholesterol-lowering fiber and bone-saving calcium, and they have a hand in protecting against colon cancer and heart disease. So instead of bagging the beans, find out which ones cause you the most trouble and boot those out of your diet. Pintos, black beans, and Great Northerns are generally the biggest gas-makers. What's gassy for some, though, may not be gassy for others. It's all a matter of how your body digests them.

If you love them but they don't love you back, there's a simple solution to eliminate most of the gas-causing effects.

1. Soak beans in water overnight.
2. Replace the water with fresh water and cook the beans for 30 minutes. Drain the water again.
3. Add fresh water and cook for another 30 minutes. Drain the water one more time.
4. Add fresh water and cook until done.

FLU (INFLUENZA)

Unlike the common cold, which causes a stuffy nose, sore throat, and sneezing, the flu is a viral infection that strikes the entire body with a vengeance. The misery starts suddenly with chills and fever and spirals into more unpleasant symptoms that will take you out of commission: a sore throat, dry cough, stuffy or runny nose, headache, nausea, vomiting, severe muscle aches and pains, weakness, backache, and loss of appetite. Some people even experience pain and stiffness in the joints.

Flu is a highly contagious illness, spread by droplets from the respiratory tract of an infected person. These can be airborne, such as those released after a person coughs or sneezes, or they can be transferred via an infected person's hands.

Taking a yearly flu shot can help you ward off infection, and these are particularly recommended for senior citizens, people with compromised immune systems, or people with asthma. They won't give you 100 percent protection, but they will significantly increase your chances of avoiding it.

If you do get the flu, there are kitchen remedies to help ease your suffering.

KITCHEN CURES

BROTH. Canned broth, whether it's beef, chicken, or vegetable, will keep you hydrated and help liquefy any mucus secretions. Broth is easy to keep down, even when you have no appetite, and will provide at least some nutrients.

HONEY. A hacking cough can keep you and every other household member up all night. Keep the peace with honey. Honey has long been used in traditional medicine for coughs. It's a simple enough recipe: Mix 1 tablespoon honey into 1 cup hot water, stir well, and enjoy. Honey acts as a natural expectorant, promoting the flow of mucus. Squeeze some lemon in if you want a little tartness.

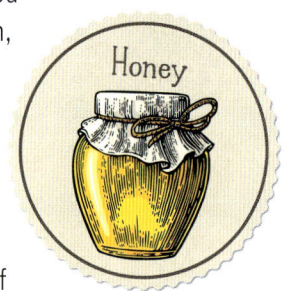

JUICE. Any flavor or kind will do. Just drink lots of juice both to keep yourself hydrated and to give yourself some extra vitamins.

LEMON. The lovely lemon may cause a puckered face if eaten raw, but in a hot beverage lemons will have you smiling. Hot lemonade has been used as a flu remedy since Roman times and is still highly regarded in the folk traditions of New England. Lemons, being highly acidic, help make mucous membranes distasteful to bacteria and viruses. Lemon oil, which gives the juice its fragrance, is like a wonder drug containing antibacterial, antiviral, antifungal, and anti-inflammatory constituents. The oil also acts as an expectorant.

PEPPER. Pepper is an irritant (try sniffling some), yet this annoying characteristic is a plus for those suffering from coughs with thick mucus. The irritating property of pepper stimulates circulation and the flow of mucus. Place 1 teaspoon black pepper into a cup and sweeten things up with the addition of 1 tablespoon honey. Fill with boiling water, let steep for 10 to 15 minutes, stir, and sip.

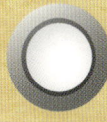

HOW TO MAKE HOT LEMONADE

To make this flu-fighting fruit drink, place 1 chopped lemon—skin, pulp, and all—into 1 cup boiling water. While the lemon steeps for 5 minutes, inhale the steam. Strain, add honey (to taste), and enjoy. Drink hot lemonade three to four times a day throughout your illness.

TEA. A cup of hot tea is just another way to take your fluids, which are so essential when you have the flu. Just be sure to choose decaffeinated varieties. Caffeine is a mild diuretic, which is counterproductive when you have the flu, and you certainly don't want to be awakened with the need to use the bathroom when you need your rest!

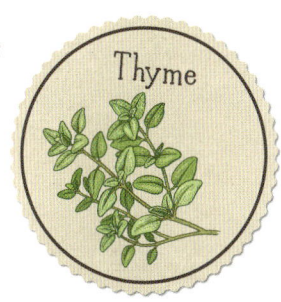

Thyme

THYME. It's time to try thyme when the mucous membranes are stuffed, the head aches, and the body is hot with fever. Wonderfully fragrant, thyme delights the senses (if you can smell when sick) and works as a powerful expectorant and antiseptic, thanks to its constituent oil, thymol. By cupping your hands around a mug of thyme tea and breathing in the steam, the thymol sets to work through your upper respiratory tract, loosening mucus and inhibiting bacteria from settling down to stay. Make thyme tea in a snap by adding 1 teaspoon dried thyme leaves to 1 cup boiling water. Let steep for five minutes while inhaling the steam. Strain the tea, sweeten with honey (to taste), and slowly sip.

FIGHT FLU WITH FLUIDS

Drink lots of fluids. Water's good, as are teas, juice, and soups. Off-limits are coffee and soda pop, as they may contain caffeine and have no nutritional benefits whatsoever.

FOOD POISONING

The symptoms you have after eating a pork chop laden with bad bacteria can range from mild (a few stomach cramps) to severe (you spend a couple of days camped out on the bathroom floor). Many people describe food poisoning as akin to being hit by a very large truck. The most common symptoms are diarrhea, stomach pain, cramping, nausea, and vomiting.

Because most of the symptoms of food poisoning are similar to those of other illnesses, such as a stomach virus, people aren't always sure food is the problem. If you think you've got food poisoning but aren't sure, take note: Most people get sick about 4 to 48 hours after eating the suspect food. And if you got sick, chances are everyone else who ate a contaminated chop will be sick, too.

FOILING FOOD POISONING

You've had some potato salad that's been sitting in the sun too long. Your stomach starts to rebel. There's not really anything you can do to stop the symptoms of food poisoning once they start, and you shouldn't try. As awful as it is, the diarrhea and vomiting that happen when you contract a foodborne illness help your body get rid of the poison. Taking over-the-counter medications that halt the process can make you sicker. The best thing you can do is take care of yourself while you're sick. These kitchen remedies can at least make dealing with the symptoms more bearable and get you feeling better faster. There are also some things in your kitchen that will help prevent food poisoning from visiting your house.

KITCHEN CURES

BANANA. As you spend more time embracing the porcelain throne, your body is losing essential elements like potassium. Losing these vital nutrients can make that I've-been-hit-by-a-truck feeling worse. Once you've come to a lull in the bathroom visitations, usually after the first 24 hours, try eating a banana. It's easy on your stomach and can make you feel a bit better.

CHICKEN SOUP. Once you start feeling a bit better, start your stomach out with bland foods. Chicken soup is tasty and easy to digest.

SPORTS DRINKS. Losing all that fluid means you're losing electrolytes (salts that keep your body functioning properly) and water. Replacing that fluid with a sports drink will help replace needed electrolytes, and the sugar in the drink will help your body better absorb the fluid it needs. If the sugar is too much for your tummy, tone the drink down by diluting it with water.

SUGAR. Sugar helps your body hold onto fluid, and adding a spoonful of sugar to a glass of water or a cup of decaffeinated tea may be more palatable if you find sports drinks too sugary.

WATER. You may not feel like having anything pass your lips, but you've got to stay hydrated, especially when you are losing fluids from both ends. Start off with a few sips of this easy-to-swallow liquid and work your way up to more substantial stuff.

MORE DO'S AND DON'TS

- Don't start back on foods that are hard to digest. Give your stomach and your intestines time to recuperate. Stay away from spicy, smoked, fried, or salty foods. Stay away from raw vegetables or rich pastries or candies, and don't drink alcohol.

- Once you're sick, get someone else to go to the kitchen for you. You could be spreading more harmful bacteria and inviting others to share in your suffering.

FOOT DISCOMFORT AND ODOR

Every day, on average, we take about 10,000 steps. That adds up to four hikes around the planet during a lifetime. And each time a step is taken, the impact of hitting the ground is about four times your body weight. No wonder, then, that 70 percent of us experience foot and ankle problems at some time.

Foot odor, known in the medical profession as bromhidrosis, can be traced to bacteria that find your moist and warm feet, socks, and shoes the perfect place to breed and multiply. Thousands of sweat glands on the soles of the feet produce perspiration composed of water, sodium chloride, fat, minerals, and various acids that are the end products of your body's metabolism. In the presence of certain bacteria (namely those found in dark, damp shoes), these sweaty secretions break down, generating the stench that turns people green.

To fight foot discomfort and odor, turn to these kitchen cures.

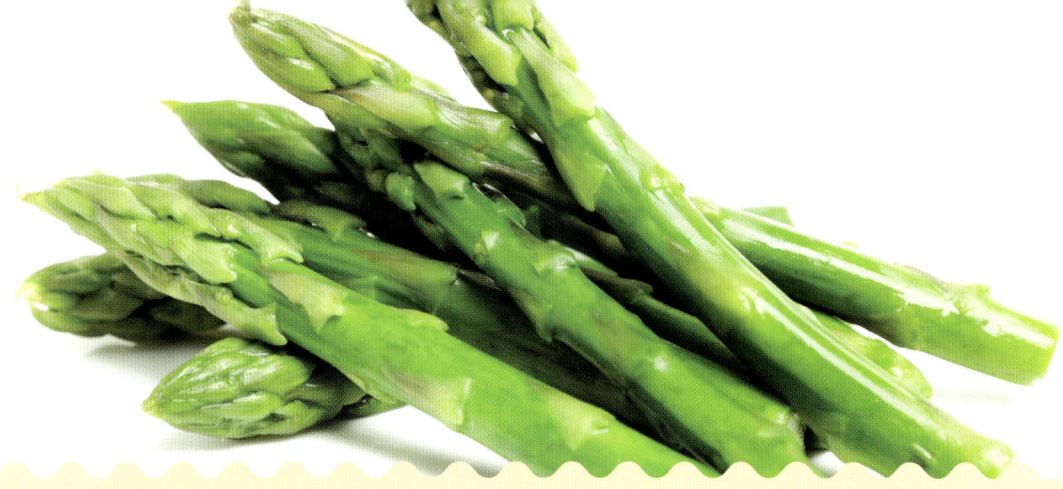

KITCHEN CURES

ASPARAGUS. For swollen feet, look in the veggie drawer for that nice, fresh asparagus you bought. Steam and eat. Asparagus acts as a natural diuretic, which flushes the excess fluid out of your system.

FOODS. For bloated, uncomfortable feet, here are some foods that can help balance your fluid levels: bananas, which are high in potassium that helps relieve fluid retention, and coffee or tea, both of which are diuretics. You can also turn to poultry and fresh fish, both of which are low in sodium, and yogurt, which can reduce histamine-producing bacteria. Histamine causes fluid retention.

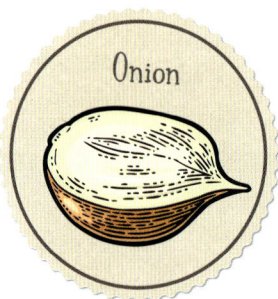

FOODS TO WATCH OUT FOR

Watch what foods you eat in abundance. Strong, pungent foods such as garlic, onions, scallions, peppers, and curry spices can cause foot odor. The odoriferous products in each pass through the bloodstream and concentrate in the perspiration.

FOODS THAT CAUSE FLUID RETENTION

Sometimes a simple dietary change is all it takes to get rid of those aching swollen feet. Avoid these foods, which can make your feet puff right up:

- Bacon and other cured meats. Curing is done with salt, which causes fluid retention.
- Lunch meats. These, too, have lots of salt.
- Canned foods. Salt is added to most canned foods, including vegetables.

GALLBLADDER PROBLEMS

Unless you've had problems with your gallbladder, you probably don't know much about it. Be thankful. If you do know the specifics of your gallbladder, you're probably one of the 10 to 15 percent of Americans who have gallstones. While half of those with gallstones experience no symptoms, the other half can have chronic problems, including discomfort and pain in the upper abdomen, indigestion, nausea, and intolerance of fatty foods. A gallbladder attack, which occurs when a gallstone gets stuck in the bile duct, can double you over in pain for hours and leave you wishing something, anything, could make you feel better.

CASTING STONES

The gallbladder is a little pear-shaped pouch tucked behind the lobes of the liver. Its main job is to store up the cholesterol-rich bile that's secreted by the liver. Bile helps your body digest fatty foods. So when that piece of prime rib reaches the intestines, they send a message up to the gallbladder to send some bile their way. Once the bile saturates your steak, it becomes more digestible and easily makes its way through the rest of the digestive process.

At least that's the way things should work. But the reality is that many people, especially older people and women, will have some gallbladder trouble. Ninety percent of the time that trouble is in the form of gallstones. Gallstones form when the bile contains excessive amounts of cholesterol. When there isn't enough bile to saturate the cholesterol, the cholesterol begins to crystallize, and you get a gallstone. These tough bits can be as tiny as a grain of sand or as large as a golf ball. You may not even know you have gallstones unless you happen to have an ultrasound or X-ray of your tummy. But the 20 percent of the time that gallstones do cause problems, it's excruciatingly painful.

Gallstones become a problem when they get pushed out of the gallbladder and into the tube that connects the liver and the small intestine. The tube gets blocked, and you get 20 minutes to 4 hours of indescribable agony. Pain usually radiates from your upper right abdominal area to your lower right chest, and it can even leave your shoulder and back in agony. Gallstones typically fall back into the gallbladder or make their way through the duct, leaving you feeling better. After you have an attack, you'll probably be sore and wonder what in the world happened.

Sometimes, though, the gallstones can get stuck in the bile duct. Symptoms of a stuck gallstone include chills, vomiting, and possibly jaundice in addition to the pain described above.

Take heart. There are some specific things you can find in your kitchen to help you avoid a gallstone attack and even prevent gallstones from forming in the first place. What you eat has a great effect on whether or not you develop gallstones. And research is finding that certain foods can help you avert a painful attack or, better yet, avoid gallstones altogether.

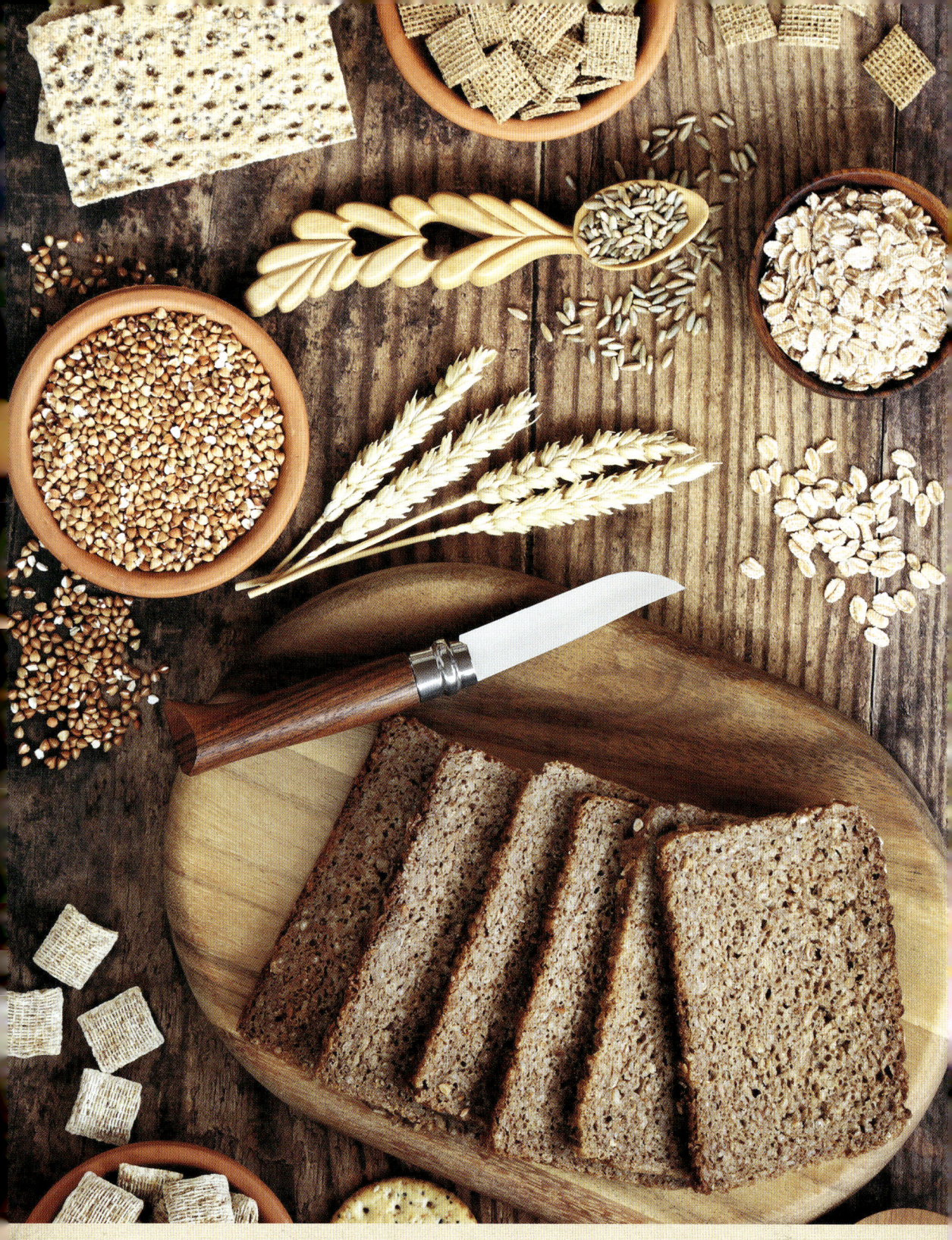

KITCHEN CURES

HIGH-FIBER CEREAL. People who eat a sugary, high-fat diet probably will have more problems with their gallstones. But adding in some fiber-rich foods and avoiding the sugary snacks and fatty foods can help you keep your gallbladder healthy. Grabbing some cereal in the morning will also get something in your tummy. Studies have shown that going for long periods without eating, such as skipping breakfast, can make you more prone to getting a gallstone.

LENTILS. An interesting study found that women who ate loads of lentils, nuts, beans, peas, lima beans, and oranges were more resistant to gallbladder attacks than women who didn't eat much of the stuff.

RED BELL PEPPER. Getting loads of vitamin C in your diet can help you avoid gallstones, and one red bell pepper has 95 mg of the helpful vitamin—more than the 60 mg a day the government recommends for men and women over age 15. A recent study found that people who had more vitamin C in their blood were less likely to get the painful stones.

Red Bell Pepper

SALMON. Research is finding that omega-3 fatty acids, found in fatty fish such as salmon, may help prevent gallstones.

VEGETABLES. Eating your veggies is a good way to ward off gallstones. One study found that vegetarian women were only half as likely to have gallstones as their carnivore counterparts. Researchers aren't sure exactly how vegetables counteract gallstones, but they believe vegetables help reduce the amount of cholesterol in bile.

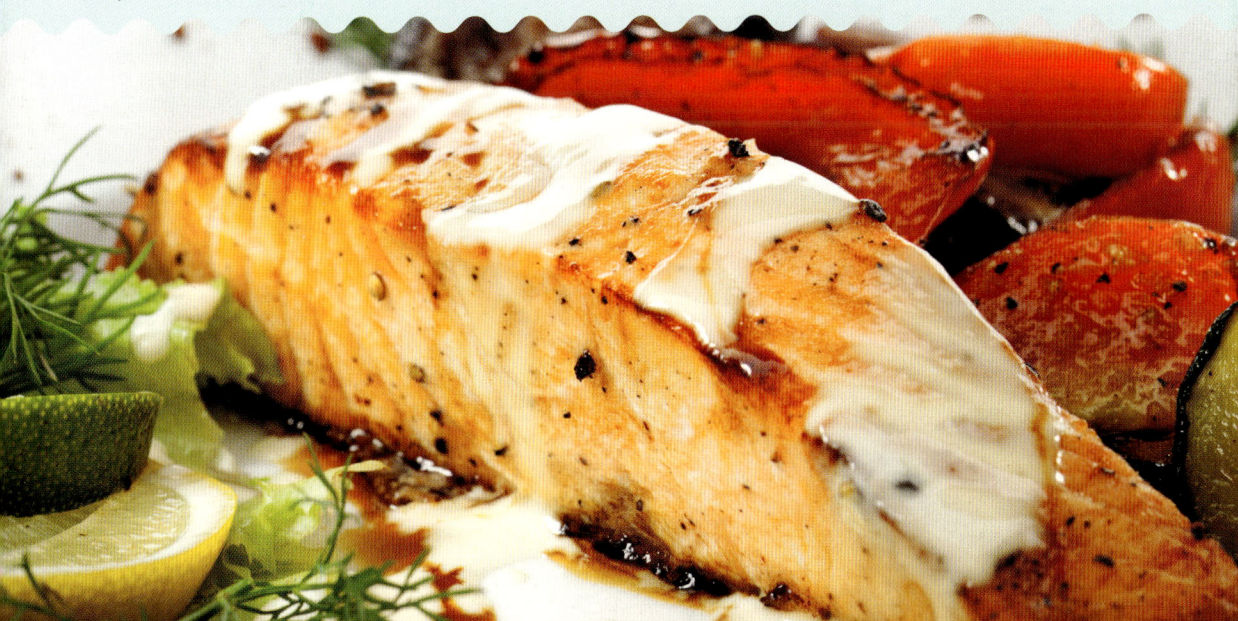

MORE DO'S AND DON'TS

- Lose some weight. Being overweight, even as little as 10 pounds, can double your risk of getting gallstones.

- Diet sensibly. If you are overweight, plan on shedding pounds slowly. Losing weight too fast can increase your chances of developing gallstones.

- Reduce your saturated fat intake. Too much fat in the diet increases your risk of gallstones. But don't cut back too drastically. You need some fat to give the gallbladder the message to empty bile. If you're trying to lose weight, don't go below 20 percent calories from fat.

- Eat a low fat, low-cholesterol, high-fiber diet. Multiple studies show this is your best bet for a healthy body and a healthy gallbladder.

GOUT

Gout, which occurs in about five percent of people with arthritis, results from the buildup of uric acid in the blood. Uric acid is the result of the breakdown of waste substances, called purines, in the body. Usually it is dissolved in the blood, processed by the kidneys, and passed out of the body in the urine. But in some people there is an excess amount of uric acid, too much for the kidneys to eliminate quickly. When there is too much uric acid in the blood, it crystallizes and collects in the joint spaces, causing gout. Occasionally, these deposits become so large that they push against the skin in lumpy patches, called tophi, that can actually be seen.

A gout attack usually lasts five to ten days, and the most common area under siege is the big toe. In fact, 75 percent of people with gout will be affected in the big toe at some time. Gout in the big toe can become so painful that even a bedsheet draped over it will cause intolerable pain. Besides the big toe, gout may also develop in the ankles, heels, knees, wrists, fingers, and elbows.

WHO GETS GOUT?

Though anyone can get gout, it's primarily a man's disease. Women have the good fortune of being more efficient in the way they excrete uric acid. And children rarely get it.

Other risk factors include:

- Family history of gout. Up to 18 percent of all people with gout have family members with gout.

- Overweight. Excessive eating steps up the production of uric acid.

- Eating too many foods with purines, such as organ meats (liver, kidney, brains, sweetbreads), sardines, anchovies, meat extracts, dried peas, lentils, and legumes.
- Heavy alcohol use.
- Exposure to environmental lead.
- Using certain medications, including diuretics, salicylates, and levodopa.
- Taking niacin, a vitamin that's also called nicotinic acid.

Gout symptoms come on quickly the first time, often overnight. You can go to bed feeling fine and wake up later in excruciating pain. You may also experience joint swelling and shiny red or purple skin around the joint. If you're already predisposed to gout, you can trigger an episode by:

- Drinking too much alcohol
- Overeating, especially purine foods
- Having surgery
- Experiencing a sudden severe illness or trauma
- Going on a crash diet
- Injuring a joint
- Having chemotherapy
- Being under stress. The link isn't the stress itself, but the comfort eating or drinking that may accompany it.

If you have gout, *professional medical treatment is required*. There are several prescription medications that are very effective at eliminating excess uric acid. Untreated, gout may progress to serious joint damage and disability. Also, excess uric acid can cause kidney stones. For gout, though, there are several kitchen remedies that can be effective along with medication to alleviate the pain and symptoms you experience.

KITCHEN CURES

APPLE PRESERVES. This may neutralize the acid that causes gout. Take as many apples as you wish, then peel, core, and slice. Simmer in a little water for three hours or more, until they turn thick, brown, and sweet. Refrigerate. Use as you would any preserve.

CELERY SEED. It neutralizes acid in the body, including the uric acid that builds up to cause gout. Crush 1 to 2 teaspoons celery seeds and place in a cup of boiling water. Steep 20 minutes, strain, then sweeten to cover the bitter taste. Drink 1 cup three times a day.

CHERRIES. Cherries may remove toxins from the body, clean the kidneys, and yes, even help give you a rosy complexion. Because of their cleansing power, they're at the top of the gout-relief list. If you can bake a cherry pie, you may be making a gout treatment. Cherry compote, cherry juice, cherry jam, cherry tea, cherry anything works.

CHICORY. If you've been to New Orleans, you know the flavor. It's in the coffee, and it's definitely an acquired taste. Chicory is an old herb, its first use recorded around the first century A.D., and over the past 2,000 years it's seen many medicinal uses. Gout is one of them. Here's a recipe said to relieve symptoms. Mix 1 ounce chicory root to 1 pint boiling water, and take as much of it as you want. This can work as a poultice, too, when it is applied to the skin in the area affected by gout.

FIGS. Crush and boil 4 figs in 1 pint water. Cook until half the water is gone. Cool, then drink.

THYME. Drink as a tea. Add 1 to 2 teaspoons to a cup of boiling water. Sweeten, and drink.

WATER. To rid yourself of uric acid, you absolutely must keep your body flushed out. Drink at least 2 quarts of water a day—more, if you can manage it.

GOOD FOODS, BAD FOODS

Diet plays an important role in gout prevention. Here are some foods that will help to keep gout under control:

- Whole-grain cereals and whole-wheat bread. These are loaded with zinc that may be depleted during a gout attack.

- Breakfast cereals and breads fortified with folic acid. These can slow the production of uric acid.

- Bread, pasta, low fat milk and dairy products, eggs, lettuce, tomatoes. These are all examples of low-purine foods.

- Citrus fruits. They have vitamin C that may assist the kidneys in ridding the body of uric acid.

And if you have gout and don't want it to come back, avoid these foods:

- Asparagus, spinach, cauliflower, mushrooms. They have purines.

- Shrimp and crabs. They also contain purines.

- Alcohol. It increases uric acid production in foods. That means beer, too!

- Dried fruit and fruit sugar. If you eat it, do so in moderation. The fructose in it produces uric acid.

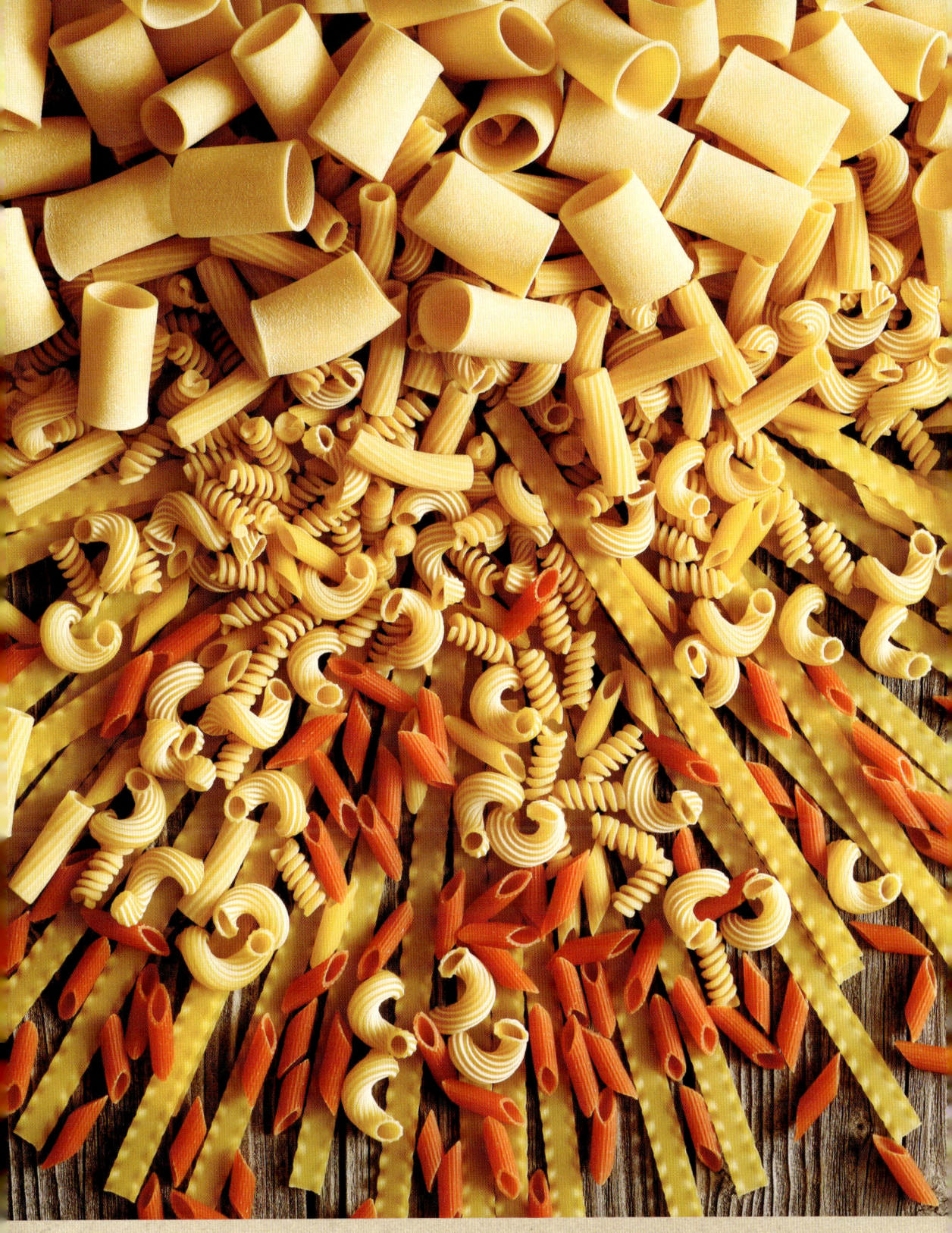

HANGOVERS

Well, you partied from sundown to sunup, and now you're paying the price. You've got the pounding headache, the queasiness, the dizziness, the sensitivity to light and sound, the muscle aches, and the irritability that comes from overconsumption of alcoholic beverages. How quickly last night's fun turns into next morning's nightmare when you have a hangover!

WHY SUCH SUFFERING?

Although we don't like to think of it as such, alcohol is actually a drug. It's a depressant, and when taken in excess, it fills your body with toxins. Your body reacts as it would to any drug overdose: It tries to metabolize and get rid of the offending substances. The debilitating symptoms you experience are a result of the body's inability to get rid of the toxins quickly enough, and they build up in your bloodstream.

Your body's attempts to flush out the alcohol puts a strain on the liver, which madly draws on the body's water reserves to get the job done. Since alcohol is a major diuretic, causing you to urinate more frequently, you lose more water than your body takes in with the beverage. As strange as it may sound, the more alcohol you drink, the more vital fluids you lose. The considerable water loss associated with drinking alcohol increases the liver's burden to get a hold of water anywhere it can. It will take water from the brain and from other vital organs. The resulting dehydration is what's behind many of the worst symptoms of a hangover.

The process of metabolizing the alcohol and excreting large quantities of water also robs the body of glucose and other vital nutrients. Being malnourished further contributes to the unpleasant hangover symptoms.

In addition to dehydration, fatigue is also behind some of your hangover pain. Excessive drinking and late nights usually go hand-in-hand. But more than that, alcohol interferes with a normal sleep pattern, robbing you of the dream state, which is essential to feeling rested. You may pass out on the floor and sleep for hours, but it won't be the kind of sleep that will allow you to restart your engines in the morning. Lack of proper rest contributes to the malaise a hangover brings.

PREVENTION

The best way to prevent a hangover is, of course, drinking in moderation or abstaining from alcohol. But keeping yourself well-hydrated and well-nourished when you're drinking can go a long way toward minimizing the morning-after symptoms. Try drinking a glass of water or other noncaffeinated beverage for each alcoholic beverage you drink. And don't drink on an empty stomach. Food helps slow the absorption of alcohol, giving your body time to metabolize it and decreasing the chances of a hangover.

The best cure for a hangover: time. Of course, people ignore the prevention and don't have "time" for the cure. So, here are some remedies to ease the suffering for those who have had one drink too many.

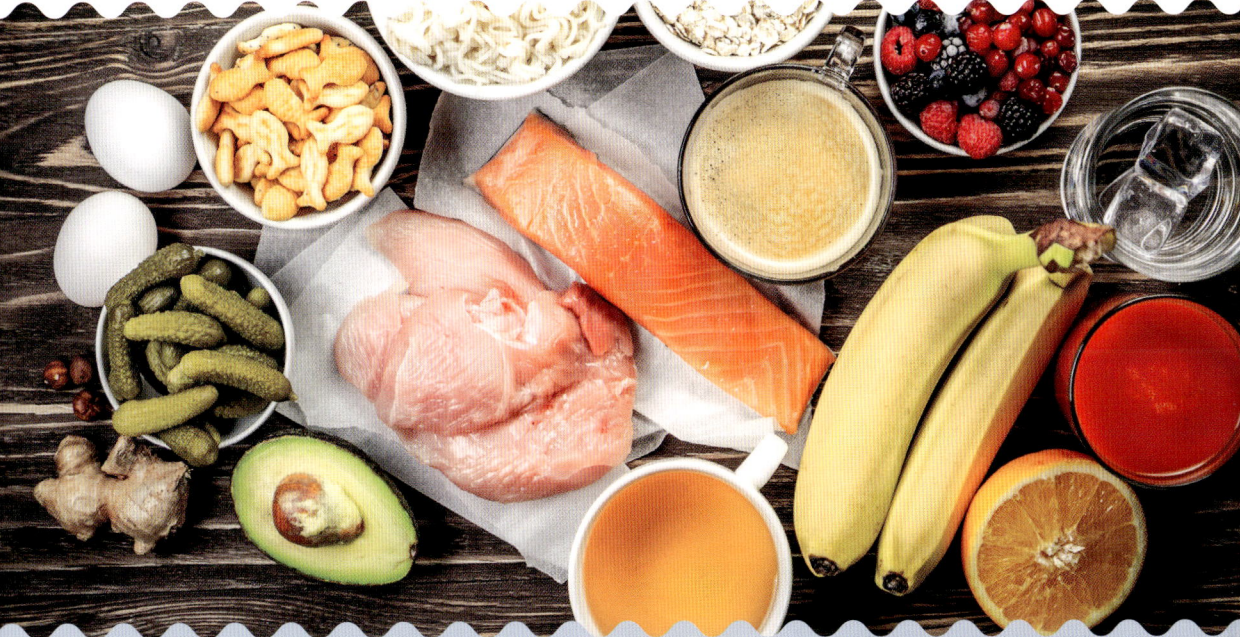

KITCHEN CURES

BANANA. Bananas are your best friend! While you were drunk and peeing like a racehorse, lots of potassium drained from your body. Eating a banana bursting with potassium will give you some giddy-up and go. All you have to do is peel and eat.

GINGER ROOT. Ginger has long been used to treat nausea and seasickness. And, since having a hangover is much like being seasick, this easy remedy works wonders. If you're really green, the best bet is to drink ginger ale (no preparation required). If you can remain vertical for ten minutes, brew some ginger tea. Cut 10 to 12 slices of fresh ginger root and combine with 4 cups water. Boil for ten minutes. Strain and add the juice of 1 orange, the juice of ½ lemon, and ½ cup honey. Drink to your relief.

JUICE. Juice, especially freshly squeezed orange juice, will help raise your blood sugar levels and help ease some of your hangover symptoms. However, if your stomach is upset, skip acidic juices such as orange juice and stick with apple juice instead.

RICE, SOUP, OR TOAST. Food is probably the last thing you want to look at while recovering, but you do need some substance for energy. Stay with clear liquids until you can tolerate something solid. Then start off slowly with mild, easy-to-digest foods such as plain toast, rice, or clear soup.

SPORTS DRINKS. These are a good way to replace fluids as well as electrolytes and glucose.

HANGOVER CURE MYTHS

Myth #1: A strong cuppa joe cures a hangover.

If only it were as easy as stopping off at Starbucks! Coffee does little, if anything, to help you sober up and may, in fact, work against you. Like alcohol, coffee is a diuretic and can further dehydrate your system. Moreover, the acidic nature of coffee can sour a sensitive stomach. What coffee can do is ease your aching headache by constricting blood vessels, but it does so at a price. Instead of brewing a cuppa, it's a better (and easier) idea to take two nonaspirin pain relievers, especially acetaminophen. Aspirin can aggravate the stomach.

Myth #2: A morning-after drink will cure a hangover.

Along the lines of the "hair-of-the-dog-that-bit-you" philosophy, drinking a glass of what you drank the night before (or any other alcohol for that matter) won't help. A morning-after drink only recreates the problem and worsens symptoms.

Myth #3: Down a big, all-American breakfast for a quick cure.

Greasy bacon, runny eggs, and fried potatoes will send you running to the toilet faster than you can say "hangover cure." The poor stomach, already irritated by alcohol, isn't prepared for this hard-to-digest, fatty trio. Give the tummy a break and stick to toast, perhaps with a little marmalade on top.

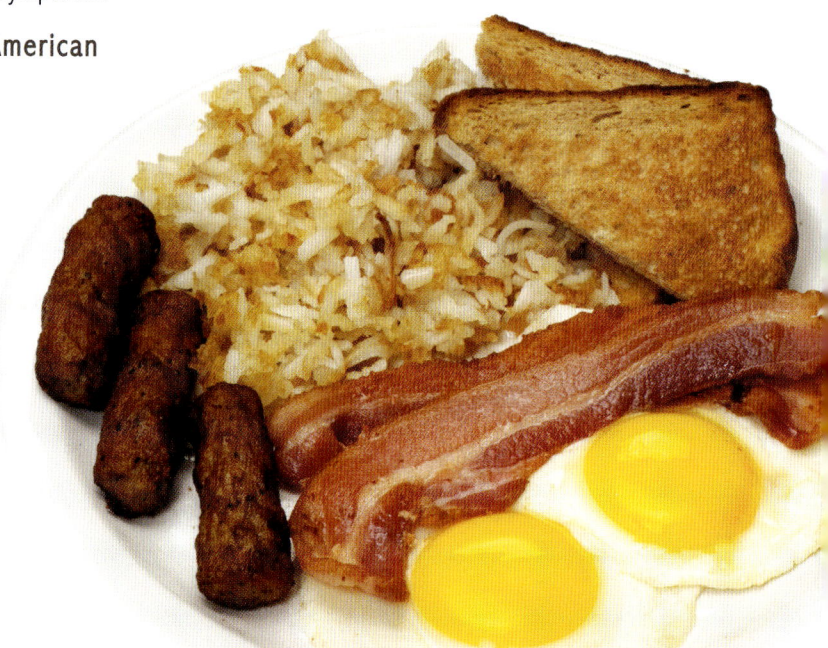

HEARTBURN

Heartburn is also known as acid indigestion. It's the feeling you get when digestive acid escapes your stomach and irritates the esophagus, the tube that leads from your throat to your stomach. After you eat, heartburn can also fire up when you bend forward, exercise, or strain muscles.

WHY ACID BACKS UP

The purpose of stomach acid is to break down the foods we eat so our body can digest them. Our stomachs have a protective lining that shields it from those acids, but the esophagus does not have that protection. Normally that's not a problem, because after we swallow food, it passes down the esophagus, through a sphincter, and into the stomach. The sphincter then closes.

Occasionally, though, the muscles of that sphincter are weakened and it doesn't close properly or it doesn't close all the way. Scarring from an ulcer or frequent episodes of acid reflux (when the acid comes back up), stomach pressure from overeating, obesity, and pregnancy can all cause this glitch in the lower esophageal sphincter (LES). And when the LES gets a glitch and allows the gastric acid to splash out of the stomach, you get heartburn.

Generally, heartburn isn't serious. In fact, small amounts of reflux are normal and most people don't even notice it because the swallowing we do causes saliva to wash the acids right back down into the stomach where they belong. When the stomach starts shooting back amounts that are larger than normal, especially on a regular basis or over a prolonged period of time, that's when the real trouble begins, and simple heartburn can turn into esophageal inflammation or bleeding.

There are several prescription medicines available for the treatment of long-term or serious heartburn or acid reflux, and over-the-counter remedies are available at your pharmacy, too. But there are several remedies right in your own kitchen that can fight the fire of heartburn.

FROM THE DRAWER

If you're prone to heartburn, keep a food diary. This can tell you which foods or food combinations cause that heartburn.

KITCHEN CURES

ALMONDS. Chewing 6 or 8 blanched almonds during an episode of heartburn may relieve the symptoms. Chew them well, though, to avoid swallowing air and causing yourself more discomfort.

APPLES. They cool the burn of stomach acid. Eat them fresh, with the skin still on, or cook them for desserts.

APPLE HONEY. This is a simple remedy that will neutralize stomach acids. Peel, core, and slice several sweet apples. Simmer with a little water over low heat for three hours until the mixture is thick, brown, and sweet to the taste. Refrigerate in an airtight container and take a few spoonfuls whenever you have the need.

BROWN RICE. Plain or with a little sweetening, rice can help relieve discomfort. Rice is a complex carbohydrate and is a bland food, which is less likely to increase acidity or relax the sphincter muscle.

BUTTERMILK. This is an acid-reliever, but don't confuse it with regular milk, which can be an acid-maker, especially if you are bothered by lactose intolerance.

CARDAMOM. This old-time digestive aid may help relieve the burn of acid indigestion. Add it to baked goodies such as sweet rolls or fruit cake, or sprinkle, with a pinch of cinnamon, on toast. It works well in cooked cereals, too.

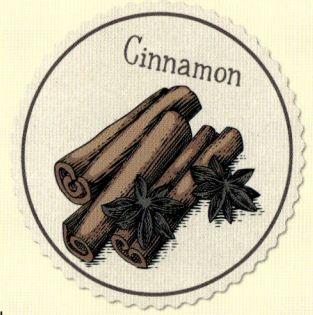

CINNAMON. This is a traditional remedy for acid relief. Brew a cup of cinnamon tea from a cinnamon stick. Or try a commercial brand, but check the label. Cinnamon tea often has black tea in it, which is a cause of heartburn, so make sure your commercial brand doesn't contain black tea. For another acid-busting treat, make cinnamon toast.

FRUIT JUICES. Skip juices from citrus fruits, but try these stomach-cooling juices for heartburn relief: papaya, mango, guava, pear.

GINGER. A tea from this root can soothe that burning belly. Add 1½ teaspoons ginger root to 1 cup water; simmer for ten minutes. Drink as needed.

LIME JUICE. Mix 10 drops lime juice with ½ teaspoon sugar and ¼ teaspoon baking soda, in that order. When the baking soda is added it will fizz, and that's when you need to drink it down. The fizz will neutralize stomach acid.

POTATO. Mix ½ cup raw potato juice with ½ cup water, and drink after meals. To make raw potato juice, simply put a peeled raw potato through a juicer or blender.

PUMPKIN. Eat it baked as a squash to get rid of heartburn. Fresh is best. Spice it up with cinnamon, which is another heartburn cure. Or, make a compote of baked pumpkin and apples, spiced with cinnamon and honey, for a dessert that's both curative and tasty.

SAGE. Use it to make a tea that can relieve stomach weakness that allows acid to be released back into the esophagus.

SODA CRACKERS. This is an old folk cure that actually works. Soda crackers (preferably unsalted) are bland, they digest easily, and they absorb stomach acid. They also contain bicarbonate of soda and cream of tartar, which neutralize the acid. Tip: You know that package of soda crackers they always give you at the restaurant, that you leave on the table? From now on, take them with you. These come in handy when you're plagued by heartburn and can't seek immediate relief.

YOGURT. Make sure it has live cultures in it. Because of the helpful and digestive-friendly microorganisms in yogurt, it may sooth the acid-forming imbalances that can lead to heartburn.

MORE DO'S & DON'TS

- Eat smaller meals. The more food in your belly, the more likely that bulk will push stomach acid right back up.

- Eat slowly, chew thoroughly. Sometimes heartburn will flare because the food is simply too large to get through the digestive tract and it, along with the acids, is forced back up.

- Don't eat right before bedtime. Give your stomach a two- or three-hour break before you sleep.

THE USUAL SUSPECTS

Here's the food list that's commonly associated with heartburn. Cut back on these, or cut them out altogether, and see what happens:

Fried and fatty foods, pies, cakes, cookies, butter, margarine, oils, cream: These may weaken your LES. Also, fatty foods take longer to digest, meaning the gastric juices are working overtime and have more opportunity to cause a backup.

Caffeinated beverages, such as coffee, tea, cola: Caffeine causes extra acid production.

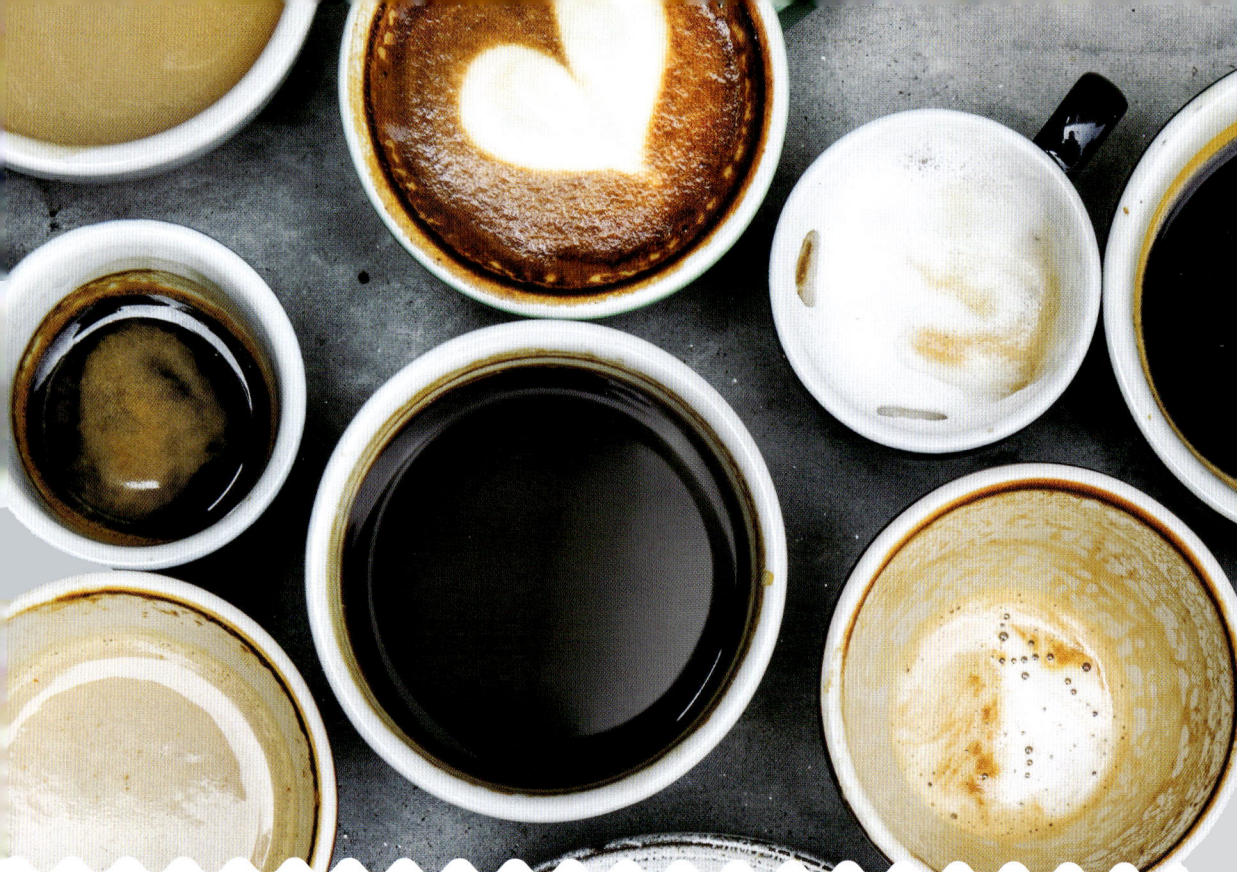

Peppermint in any form*: It relaxes the stomach muscle and valve, allowing the release of acids back up into the esophagus.

Chocolate: It contains methylxanthines, a second cousin to caffeine, and can weaken the stomach valve.

Fruit and vegetable juices, especially tomato and citrus juice: They can irritate the throat and cause pain if heartburn has already caused irritation. Pineapple juice has an especially potent punch.

Garlic and onions: May weaken the LES.

Spicy, pickled, or fermented foods: These are heartburn-makers, too.

Alcohol: It causes the LES to relax.

Smoking and certain drugs such as aspirin, ibuprofen, and some antibiotics: These also relax the LES, causing acid reflux.

**Warning!* Peppermint is often prescribed for other symptoms of indigestion but should never be used when heartburn is present.

HEART DISEASE

Heart disease is any condition that keeps your heart from functioning at its best or causes a deterioration of the heart's arteries and vessels. Coronary heart disease (CHD), also known as coronary artery disease, is the most common form of heart disease. If you are diagnosed with CHD, it means you have atherosclerosis, or hardening of the arteries on the heart's surface. Arteries become hard when plaque accumulates on artery walls. This plaque develops gradually as an overabundance of low-density lipoprotein (LDL) cholesterol (the bad stuff) makes itself at home in your arteries. The plaque builds and narrows the artery walls, making it more and more difficult for blood to pass through the heart and increasing the opportunity for a blood clot to form. If the heart doesn't get enough blood, it can cause chest pain (angina) or a heart attack.

There are many risk factors for heart disease, some you can do something about, and some you can't. A family history of heart disease puts you at much greater risk for developing it yourself. Your best strategies for fighting heart disease will be developed by you and your medical team. But you can find help in food as well.

KITCHEN CURES

BRAN. Bran cereal is a high-fiber food that will help keep your cholesterol levels in check. Other high fiber foods in your cupboard include barley, oats, whole grains such as brown rice and lentils, and beans, such as kidney beans and black beans.

BROCCOLI. Calcium is another heart-healthy nutrient, and milk isn't the only calcium-rich food. In fact, there are lots of nondairy foods that are rich in calcium, such as kale, salmon, figs, pinto beans, and okra. One cup of broccoli can supply you with 90 mg of calcium.

CHICKEN. Three ounces of chicken will give you ⅓ of your daily requirement for vitamin B6, a necessary nutrient for maintaining your heart health.

GARLIC. Chock-full of antioxidants, garlic seems to be able to lessen plaque buildup, reduce the incidence of chest pain, and keep the heart generally healthy. It is also a mild anticoagulant, helping to thin the blood. The advantages may take some time: One study found that it took a couple of years of eating garlic daily to get its heart-healthy benefits.

OLIVE OIL. The American Heart Association and the American Dietetic Association recommend getting most of your fat from monounsaturated sources. Olive oil is a prime candidate. Try using it instead of other vegetable oils when sautéing your veggies.

PEANUT BUTTER. Eat 2 tablespoons of this comforting food and you can get ⅓ of your daily intake of vitamin E. Because vitamin E is a fat-soluble vitamin (other antioxidant vitamins are water soluble), it is found more abundantly in fattier foods like vegetable oils and nuts. If you're watching your weight, don't go overboard on the peanut butter.

PECANS. These tasty nuts are full of magnesium, another heart-friendly nutrient. One ounce of pecans drizzled over a spinach salad can give you ⅓ of your recommended daily allowance of this vital mineral.

SALMON. Adding fatty fish to your diet is a good idea if you're at risk for heart disease. Three ounces of salmon meets your daily requirement for vitamin B12, a vitamin that helps keep your heart healthy, and it's a good source of omega-3 fatty acids, which have been proven to lower triglycerides and reduce blood clots that could potentially block arteries in the heart.

SPINACH. Make yourself a salad using spinach instead of the usual iceberg lettuce and get a good start on meeting your folic acid needs (½ cup has 130 mcg of folic acid). Along with the other B vitamins, B6 and B12, folic acid can help prevent heart disease.

STRAWBERRIES. Oranges aren't the only fruit loaded with vitamin C. You can fill up on 45 milligrams of the heart healthy vitamin with ½ cup of summer's sweet berry. Vitamin C is an antioxidant vital to maintaining a happy heart. Strawberries are also a good source of fiber and potassium, both important to heart health.

SWEET POTATOES. With double your daily requirements for vitamin A, a heart-protecting nutrient, sweet potatoes are a smart choice for fending off heart disease.

WHOLE-WHEAT BREAD. Slather some peanut butter on a slice of whole-wheat bread and you've got a snack that's good to your heart. One slice of whole-wheat bread has 11 mcg of selenium, an antioxidant mineral that works with vitamin E to protect your heart.

HIGH BLOOD PRESSURE

Sometimes what you don't know can hurt you. Such is the case with high blood pressure, or hypertension. Although one in four adults has high blood pressure, according to the American Heart Association (AHA), almost a third of them don't know they have it.

That's because high blood pressure often has no symptoms. It's not as if you feel the pressure of your blood coursing through your circulatory system. When the heart beats, it pumps blood to the arteries, creating pressure within them. That pressure can be normal or it can be excessive. High blood pressure is defined as a persistently elevated pressure of blood within the arteries.

Over time, the excessive force exerted against the arteries damages and scars them. It can also damage organs, such as the heart, kidneys, and brain. High blood pressure can lead to strokes, blindness, kidney failure, and heart failure.

In 90 to 95 percent of all cases, the cause of high blood pressure isn't known. In such cases, when there is no underlying cause, the disease is known as primary, or essential, hypertension. Sometimes the high blood pressure is caused by another disease, such as an endocrine disorder. In such cases the disease is called secondary hypertension.

The key to controlling high blood pressure is knowing you have it. Under the guidance of a physician, you can battle hypertension through diet, exercise, lifestyle changes, and medication, if necessary. The kitchen holds several blood pressure helpers.

KITCHEN CURES

BANANAS. The banana has been proved to help reduce blood pressure. The average person needs three to four servings of potassium-rich fruits and vegetables each day. Some experts believe doubling this amount may benefit your blood pressure. If bananas aren't your favorite bunch of fruit, try dried apricots, raisins, currants, orange juice, spinach, boiled potatoes with skin, baked sweet potatoes, cantaloupe, and winter squash.

BREADS. Be good to your blood with a bit more "B," as in the B vitamin folate. Swimming around the blood is a substance called homocysteine, which at high levels is thought to reduce the stretching ability of the arteries. If the arteries are stiff as a board, the heart pumps extra hard to move the blood around. Folate helps reduce the levels of homocysteine, in turn helping arteries become pliable. You'll find folate in fortified breads and cereals, asparagus, Brussels sprouts, and beans.

BROCCOLI. This vegetable is high in fiber, and a high fiber diet is known to help reduce blood pressure. So indulge in this and other fruits and vegetables that are high in fiber.

CANOLA, MUSTARD SEED, OR SAFFLOWER OILS. Switching to polyunsaturated oils can make a big difference in your blood pressure readings. Switching to them will also reduce your blood cholesterol level.

CAYENNE PEPPER. This fiery spice is a popular home treatment for mild high blood pressure. Cayenne pepper allows smooth blood flow by preventing platelets from clumping together and accumulating in the blood. Add some cayenne pepper to salt-free seasonings, or add a dash to a salad or in salt-free soups.

Cayenne Pepper

CELERY. Because it contains high levels of 3-N-butylphthalide, a phytochemical that helps lower blood pressure, celery is in a class by itself. This phytochemical is not found in most other vegetables. Celery may also reduce stress hormones that constrict blood vessels, so it may be most effective in those whose high blood pressure is the result of mental stress.

MILK. The calcium in milk does more than build strong bones; it plays a modest role in preventing high blood pressure. Be sure to drink skim milk or eat low fat yogurt. Leafy green vegetables also provide calcium.

SALT WEARS MANY DISGUISES

Lose the saltshaker. Although there is some debate about salt's role in high blood pressure, most experts agree that cutting back on salt intake can reduce blood pressure. Sodium chloride isn't the only name for salt. Soda or sodium also indicate the presence of salt. Look closely at labels for these sources of salt.

- Monosodium glutamate (MSG) is a popular flavor enhancer in restaurant cooking and in packaged and canned foods and seasoning mixes.

- Baking soda (sodium bicarbonate or bicarbonate of soda) and baking power are often used to leaven breads and cakes.

- Disodium phosphate is found in some quick-cooking cereals and processed cheeses.

EATING FRESH

If you have high blood pressure or are at risk for it, skip processed foods. Not only are they loaded with sodium (salt) but they are also high in saturated (read: artery-clogging) fat. Read labels, as it's not always obvious which foods contain the most sodium and saturated fat.

- Sodium alginate is what makes ice cream smooth.

- Sodium benzoate is used as a preservative in many condiments.

- Sodium hydroxide is used to soften and loosen skins of ripe olives and certain fruits and vegetables.

- Sodium nitrate is used to cure meats and sausages.

- Sodium propionate helps inhibit the growth of molds in baked goods.

- Sodium sulfite is used to bleach foods that will then be colored or glazed. It's also used as a preservative in some dried fruits.

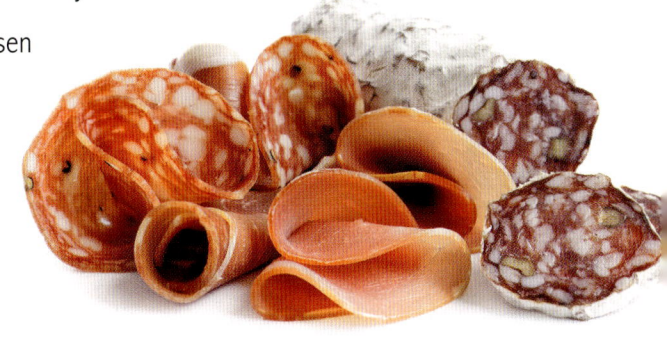

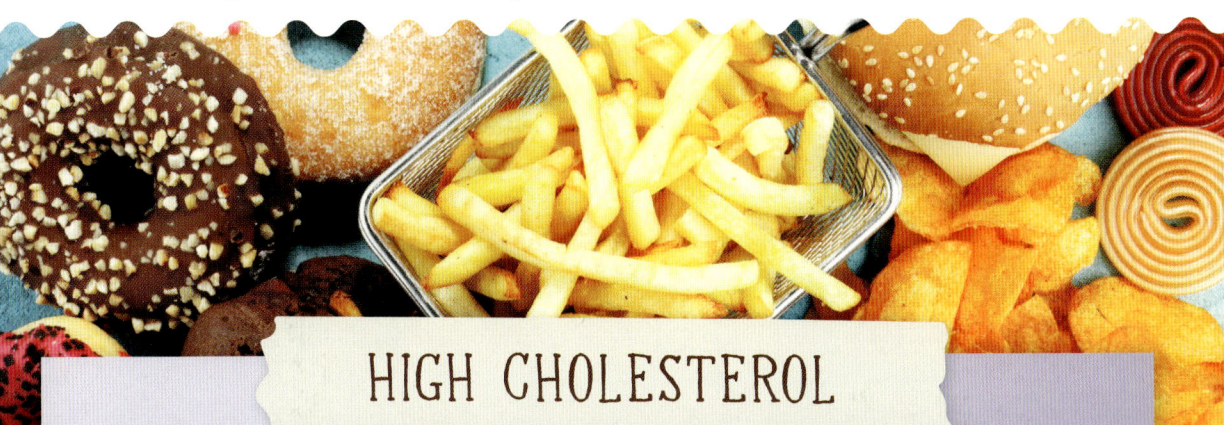

HIGH CHOLESTEROL

Cholesterol is that waxy, soft stuff that floats around in your bloodstream as well as in all the cells in your body. It takes a bad rap these days because the word *cholesterol* strikes fear in the hearts of even the healthiest of people.

Having cholesterol in your blood is normal and even healthy because it's used in the formation of cell membranes, tissues, and essential hormones. So, in proper amounts, cholesterol is good. In excessive amounts, though, it can clog the arteries leading to your heart and cause coronary disease, heart attack, or stroke.

Cholesterol comes from two sources: the foods you eat and your very own liver. And the truth of the matter is, your liver can produce all the cholesterol your body will ever need. This means that what you get in your food isn't necessary. Some people get rid of extra cholesterol easily through normal bodily waste mechanisms, but others hang on to it because their bodies just aren't as efficient in removing it, which puts them at risk.

GOOD AND BAD CHOLESTEROL?

There are two different kinds of cholesterol, and yes, one's good and one's bad. Cholesterol can't get around on its own, so it hitches a ride from lipoproteins to get to the body's cells. Problem is, there are two different rigs picking it up: One is called HDL, or high-density lipoprotein, the other is called LDL, or low-density lipoprotein. HDL is the good ride; it travels away from your arteries. LDL is the bad ride; it heads straight to your arteries. Bottom line: HDL is what you want more of; you want less of LDL.

High cholesterol can be cured two ways: by medication and/or by diet. There are numerous effective drugs on the market that will make drastic reductions in cholesterol levels, but they all come with side effects and require frequent blood tests to monitor for possible problems. But there are kitchen cures, and they may work on their own or along with conventional treatment. Whatever your cure, it must come with advice from your doctor since your heart is at risk.

KITCHEN CURES

ALFALFA SPROUTS. These may improve or normalize cholesterol levels.

Warning! Sprouts are not clean or washed when you buy them in the store, and they may be a source of *E.coli* bacteria. Wash thoroughly before you consume or use a veggie-cleaning product available in most grocery stores.

ALMONDS. Studies indicate that snacking on almonds regularly for as little as three weeks may decrease LDL by up to ten percent.

APPLES. Apples are high in pectin, which can lower cholesterol levels.

ARTICHOKES. This veggie can actually lower cholesterol levels. Early studies pointed to their beneficial cholesterol-busting properties, but recent studies have shown that artichokes may be even more effective than they were first thought to be.

BEETS. Full of carotenoids and flavonoids, beets help lower—and may even prevent—the formation of LDL, the bad cholesterol.

CARROTS. Full of pectin, they're as good as apples in lowering cholesterol levels.

GARLIC. Studies show that garlic may not only reduce LDL but raise HDL and decrease the amount of fat in your blood. Add some fresh garlic regularly to your cooking to keep your heart healthy.

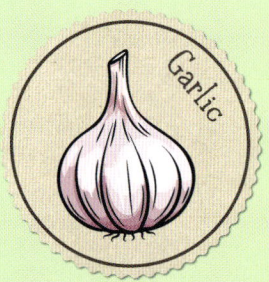

HONEY. Add 1 teaspoon honey to 1 cup hot water in the morning, and you may rid your system of excess fat and cholesterol, according to Ayurvedic medicine. Add 1 teaspoon lime juice or 10 drops cider vinegar to give that drink a more powerful cholesterol-fighting punch.

OATS. In any pure form, oats are a traditional cholesterol buster. Eating only ½ cup oatmeal a day, along with a low fat diet, may reduce cholesterol levels by nine percent.

OLIVE OIL. It protects your heart by lowering LDL, raising HDL, and preventing your blood from forming clots.

PEARS. These are high in soluble fiber, which helps regulate cholesterol levels.

RHUBARB. Yep, this is a cholesterol-buster. Consume it after a meal that's heavy in fats. You can cook it in a double boiler, with a little honey or maple syrup for added sweetness, until done. Add cardamom or vanilla if you like.

RICE. The oil that comes from the bran of rice is known to lower cholesterol. And brown rice is particularly high in fiber, which is essential in a cholesterol-lowering diet. One cup provides 11 percent of the daily fiber requirement.

SOYBEANS. These beauties may reduce LDL by as much as 20 percent when 25 to 50 grams of soy protein are eaten daily for as short a time as a month. Besides that obvious benefit, soy may fend off a rise in LDL in people with normal levels and also improve the ability of arteries to dilate. This means they expand better to allow the unimpeded passage of fats and other substances that otherwise might cause a blockage.

TURMERIC. This may lower blood cholesterol. Added to eggplant, you may reap twice the cholesterol-fighting benefit. Mix ¾ teaspoon turmeric with 2 tablespoons cooked, mashed eggplant and 1½ tablespoons boiling water. Spread it on whole wheat bread and eat after a meal heavy in fats.

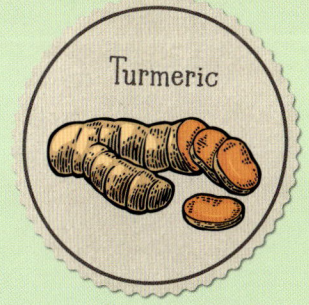

WALNUTS. A cholesterol-lowering diet that includes walnuts eaten at least four times a week may lower LDL by as much as 16 percent. And studies indicate that those who munch on these nuts regularly cut their risk of death by heart attack in half when compared to non-walnut munchers.

YOGURT. Eating 1 cup plain yogurt with active cultures a day may reduce LDL by four percent or more and total cholesterol by at least three percent. Some scientists believe that eating yogurt regularly may even reduce the overall risk of heart disease by as much as ten percent.

MORE DO'S & DON'TS

- Don't grease those pans. Use a nonstick olive oil spray or buy an inexpensive oil mister in a kitchenware store and make your own spray.

- Bulk up. Whole grains are high in fiber. Stick to complex carbohydrates, too, because they fill you up faster and leave you feeling satisfied. Try eating more fruits, veggies, pasta, rice.

- Read the food labels. They list the cholesterol content, so keep your cholesterol goal in mind: less than 300 mg a day.

- Eat small meals. Instead of 3 big meals a day, go for 5 or 6 small meals. The body deals with cholesterol intake more efficiently when it comes in small amounts.

FAT FACT

The more liquid the margarine (tub, liquid form), the less hydrogenated it is and the less trans fatty acid it contains. Trans fatty acids raise total blood cholesterol levels, so the less of them you eat, the better off you are.

INSOMNIA

Insomnia can be classified in one of three ways—trouble falling asleep (called sleep-onset insomnia), trouble staying asleep (called sleep-maintenance insomnia), or waking up feeling groggy and sleepy after what should have been a full night's sleep. Most episodes of insomnia last anywhere from a couple of nights to a few weeks. There are myriad causes, including stress, anxiety, depression, disease, pain, medications, or simply not creating a relaxing sleep routine.

There's no magic number when it comes to how many hours you should sleep. Some people get by just fine on a few hours, and some people need more than eight. But it won't be a mystery to you if you're not getting enough sleep. Waking up exhausted and being sleepy most of the day are signs that you're not well-rested.

RESTLESS LEGS

Restless legs syndrome is a frustrating condition. The name of the problem explains it all. When you finally get into bed, your legs decide it's time to get up and move. The symptoms of restless legs syndrome have been described as tingling, crawling, or prickling sensations that peak during times of inactivity, such as when you're trying to go to sleep. Walking, massaging your legs, or taking a hot shower can help relieve the problem for a bit, but it'll come back, leaving you with a sleep-deprived night. Restless legs syndrome has been connected with a deficiency in iron and folic acid. The problem worsens with age and is more frequently diagnosed in people over 65. It can be treated with prescription medicines.

INSOMNIA'S ILL EFFECTS

Insomnia can have a significant impact on your health and well-being. If you don't get enough sleep, you're setting yourself up for some serious problems. People with insomnia are

- Four times more likely to be diagnosed with depression.
- More likely to have a serious illness, including heart disease.
- More likely to have an accident on the job, at home, or on the road.
- More likely to miss work and accomplish less on the job than well-rested coworkers.

Fortunately, you can find some relief in food.

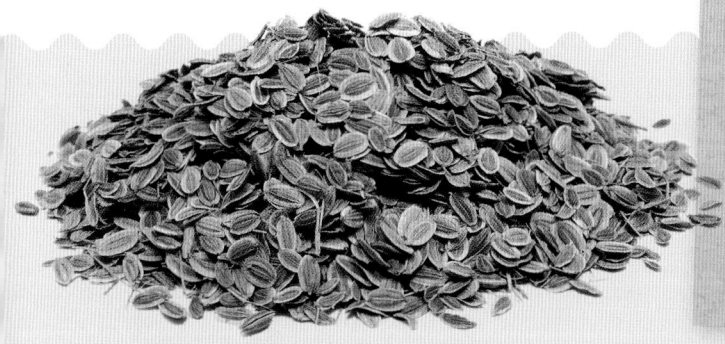

DRINKS TO AVOID

- Cut out the caffeine. Caffeine, by its nature, stimulates your brain. When you're trying to snooze, caffeine can cause problems. Having a couple of cups of coffee or a soda early in the day is fine, but switch to decaf after lunch.
- Avoid alcohol. Yes, alcohol is a sedative, but the effects soon wear off and you'll end up tossing and turning.

KITCHEN CURES

DILL SEED. Though scientists haven't proved its worth, this herb is often used as a folk cure for insomnia in China. Its essential oil has the most sedative-producing properties.

HONEY. Folk remedies often advise people with sleeping difficulty to eat a little honey. It has the same sedative effect as sugar and may get you to bed more quickly. Try adding 1 tablespoon honey to some decaffeinated herbal tea or even to your warm milk for a relaxing pre-sleep drink.

MILK. Drinking a glass of milk, especially a glass of warm milk, before bedtime is an age-old treatment for sleeping troubles. There is some debate, however, about what it is in milk—if anything—that helps cause slumber. Some scientists believe it's the presence of tryptophan, a chemical that helps the brain ease into sleep mode, that does the trick. Others believe it may be another ingredient, a soothing group of opiatelike chemicals called casomorphins. Whatever the reason, milk seems to help some people hit the sack more easily. And warm milk seems to be more effective at relaxing body and mind. Other foods high on the tryptophan scale are cottage cheese, cashews, chicken, turkey, soybeans, and tuna.

TOAST. High carbohydrate, low-protein bedtime snacks can make sleeping easier. Carbohydrate-rich foods tend to be easy on the tummy and can ease the brain into blissful slumber.

HERBS THAT HELP YOU SLEEP

Sleep problems have been around since biblical times, so it's no wonder that there are many, many botanical remedies for insomnia. Here are a few of the most common.

CHAMOMILE. Chamomile tea is one of the most popular sleep-inducing drinks on the market. It's been used in folk medicine for years and is best used for sleep problems due to upset stomach. To brew your own chamomile tea: Put 1 heaping tablespoon chamomile flowers in a cup. Add boiling water, cover, and let steep for ten minutes.

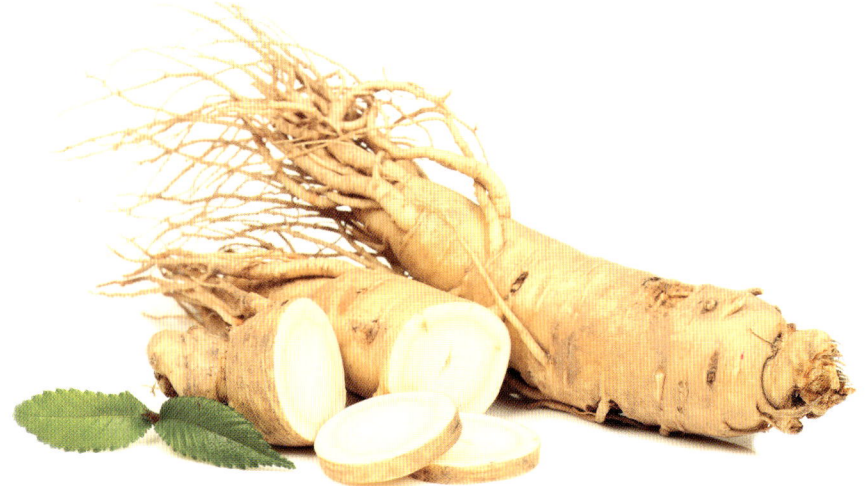

GINSENG. Drinking a ginseng wine may help sleepless nights, especially if they're related to stress or a fever-producing illness. Chop 3½ ounces ginseng (use only American ginseng) and place in 1 quart liquor, such as vodka. Let it stand for five to six weeks in a cool, dark place. Turn the container frequently. Take 1 ounce before bed.

LAVENDER. The scent of lavender is so calming that in one study it was actually as potent as a tranquilizer. In Germany, where herbs are prescribed for medical conditions, doctors often give lavender for insomnia. You can find lavender essential oil at natural food stores.

IRRITABLE BOWEL SYNDROME

You're enjoying the evening, having a nice meal at a nice restaurant, feeling pretty good. Coffee and dessert come and you're lingering over pleasant conversation, then all of a sudden wham! Out of the blue you've got a belly cramp. And suddenly you're off to find the nearest facility. There was no warning, no nothing. It just hit, and now your evening is on hold, changed, or canceled until you see how this latest attack resolves itself.

Irritable Bowel Syndrome (IBS) is a real condition, with real symptoms. But it's a mysterious one to medical experts, who still don't know what it is or what causes it exactly. What they do know is that it's common—about 15 percent of all adults are afflicted with it sometime in their lives—and that it is a malfunction of the digestive tract.

Symptoms of irritable bowel syndrome include:

- Diarrhea or constipation, or alternate bouts of each
- Abdominal pain or cramping
- Gas and bloating
- Nausea, especially after eating
- Headache
- Fatigue
- Depression or anxiety
- Mucus-covered stools
- The urge to have another bowel movement after you've just had one

IBS AND YOU

Keep a food diary and track the foods that seem to trigger the attacks. Eliminate a specific food for a couple of weeks to see if that makes a difference. If it does, you may have isolated the cause. If not, go back to your food diary, then choose another food you've eaten around the time of an attack and eliminate it. This is called an exclusion diet, and if what you're eating is a trigger for IBS, this is the best way to find out what it is. Also make note of anxiety or stress you're feeling and what you think is causing it. If you notice that your attacks seem to come during stressful events, you may need to consider ways to eliminate them.

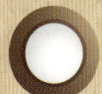

Conditions 151

WHAT WE KNOW

Irritable bowel syndrome is also called spastic colon. It's an apt name that describes the abnormal digestive function that's typical of IBS. Normally, food is pushed through the intestine by synchronized muscle contractions. They are all dancing the same dance. But then something happens and one of those dancers steps out of the chorus line, does its own dance, and messes up everybody else's rhythm. As a result, the food that's being passed down that chorus line is suddenly disrupted in its travel.

IBS is frustrating and inconvenient, but it's not serious, even though it does stand shoulder to shoulder with the common cold as a major reason for people to miss work. But the good news is, IBS doesn't lead to other more serious intestinal conditions. And it can be treated with medications that relieve the symptoms. However, treatment isn't always easy, since the cause isn't known.

Regardless of the source of the problem, it does seem that there are some remedies for IBS symptoms right in your own kitchen.

KITCHEN CURES

CABBAGE. Juice of the cabbage soothes the symptoms of intestinal ills. To turn this veggie into juice, simply wash and put through a juicer or blender. If these are not available to you, cook the cabbage in a very small amount of water—just enough to keep it from scorching or burning—until very mushy. Then pulverize with a fork or mixer.

CARROTS. These little gems help prevent the symptoms of IBS as well as regulate diarrhea and constipation. Eat them raw, by themselves or in salads, or eat them cooked—steamed and tossed with a little melted butter and brown sugar for a sweet treat. You can put raw carrots through the juicer, too. Since they're not a juicy veggie to begin with, add a little pure apricot nectar when you make carrot juice. Any way you eat a carrot is fine, just don't overcook them so much that you boil out all the goodness.

FENNEL SEEDS. These can relieve the intestinal spasms associated with IBS. They may also aid in the elimination of fats from the digestive system, inhibiting the over-production of mucus in the intestine, which is a symptom of the ailment. Steep the seeds into a tea by adding ½ teaspoon fennel to 1 cup boiling water. Or add them to veggies such as carrots or cabbage, both of which soothe IBS symptoms. You can also sprinkle the seeds on salads or roast them and snack on them after a meal to reduce the symptoms of IBS and freshen your breath. To roast, spritz a baking sheet with olive oil, then cover with fennel seeds. Bake at 325°F for 10 to 15 minutes.

FLAXSEED. Make a tea using 1 teaspoon flaxseed per cup of water, and drink at bedtime for relief of symptoms.

LETTUCE. You can eat it raw to relieve symptoms of IBS, but it's especially helpful if lightly steamed. And when you're picking out your lettuce, go for the darker varieties. The darker the color, the more nutrients it contains.

OAT BRAN. Increasing fiber is a cure for almost every intestinal ill, and oat bran is especially good for IBS because it's mild and usually colon-friendly. So use some every day: a bowl of oatmeal, oat bran bread, oatmeal cookies. But don't expect immediate results. It may take up to a month to get any IBS relief.

PEARS. Fresh, ripe, sweet pears are a nutritious fruit that also helps relieve the symptoms of IBS. Buy them when they're still hard and let them ripen at room temperature for a few days. Pure pear juice and dried pears are also helpful in treating this intestinal woe.

PEPPERMINT. Steeped into a nice, relaxing tea, this can relieve intestinal spasms. Use 1 heaping teaspoon dried peppermint, and steep in 1 cup boiling water for ten minutes. Drink as often as necessary.

YOGURT. Yogurt with active cultures will supply your digestive tract with the helpful kind of bacteria, which can ease IBS symptoms. You can also try mixing 1 cup yogurt with ½ teaspoon psyllium husks (or psyllium bulk you can buy in any pharmacy) and eating the mixture one hour after meals.

MORE DO'S & DON'TS

- Make sure you get enough fiber. It helps maintain good bowel function. You need about 35 grams a day. Chances are you're only getting about half of what you need.

- Limit alcohol and caffeine. They irritate your stomach lining, which can lead to IBS symptoms.

- Nix the tobacco. It can cause stomach cramps, among other deadly things.

- Skip the gassy foods. And try to eliminate air swallowing. The more gas you introduce into your intestine, the more likely a flare-up of IBS.

- Drink between meals, not with meals. Drinking when you eat dilutes digestive juices and frustrates digestion.

- Avoid anything that causes stress. Relax during mealtimes. Give yourself plenty of time to complete your tasks. Avoid the morning rush-rush hassle by getting up a few minutes earlier. Spend a few minutes alone, working on progressive relaxation.

NO-NO FOODS

You may have your own personal list of foods that cause your IBS flare-ups, but these are a common cause, too:

- Dairy products
- Cereals, especially wheat cereals
- Red kidney beans
- Lentils
- Peas
- Apples
- Grapes
- Raisins
- Brussels sprouts
- Broccoli
- Cauliflower
- Preserved, processed, or cured meats

LACTOSE INTOLERANCE

Lactose, the milk sugar in dairy products, can be pretty rough to digest on a good day. But our bodies manage to do it with the help of an enzyme called lactase that breaks down those tough milk sugars and converts them into glucose, or blood sugar. When lactase kicks in, milk digestion comes off without a hitch.

When there is an insufficient amount of lactase, your condition is called lactose intolerance, and it can cause some pretty miserable symptoms. Instead of being broken down, lactose instead stays intact in the intestines, absorbing fluids. When this happens, gas, cramping, heartburn, and diarrhea can result one by one or all together.

To add insult to injury, certain bacteria that call the colon home ferment the undigested lactose, causing more gas, cramping, and diarrhea.

Most adults who are lactose intolerant usually tolerated small amounts of lactose when they were children. With aging, however, the ability to digest lactose diminishes, even for those who aren't lactose intolerant. To some degree, lactose intolerance develops in virtually everyone as they age.

One way to get some idea of whether you're lactose intolerant is simply to avoid all dairy products for several weeks and see if your symptoms resolve. This isn't a conclusive method, as there may be other reasons that your symptoms don't entirely disappear. But if your symptoms do decrease, you will benefit by decreasing dairy in your diet, using a dietary aid that replaces lactase (available in most pharmacies), or using a lactose-free milk product.

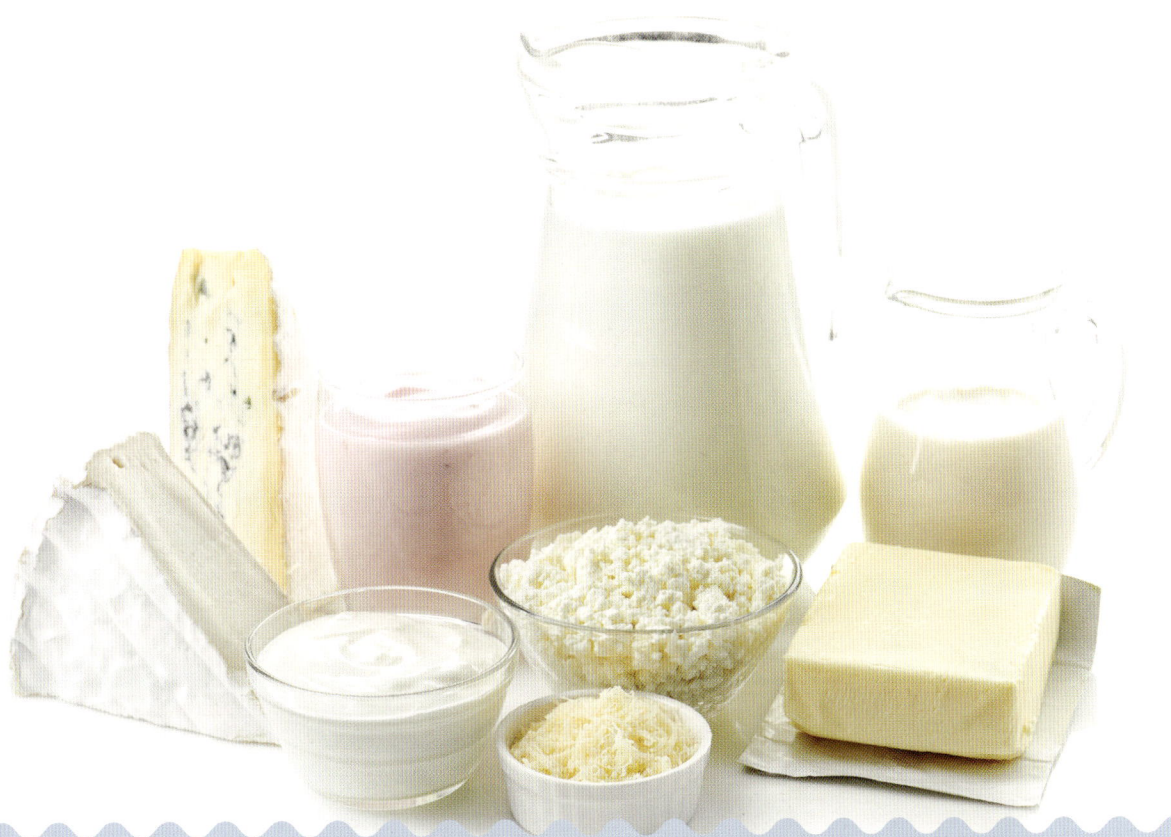

KITCHEN CURES

BUTTERMILK. It's more digestible than regular cow's milk. So is goat's milk.

COCOA POWDER. Studies indicate that cocoa powder and sugar, or chocolate powders, may help the body digest lactose by slowing the rate at which the stomach empties. The slower the emptying process, the less lactose that enters your system at once. That means fewer symptoms.

HARD CHEESE. Cheddar and Colby are good: The harder the cheese, the lower its lactose content. Skip the soft cheese, including cream cheese, cottage cheese, and any product that's processed or spreadable.

MILK. People with any degree of lactose intolerance should never drink milk by itself. Always have a snack with your milk or have it with a meal.

SARDINES. They're high in calcium, which might be lacking in your diet if you're not drinking milk or consuming calcium-rich milk products. These foods are also high in calcium: canned salmon (or any other canned oily fish with bones), tofu, dark green leafy vegetables, nuts, cooked dried beans, dried apricots, and sesame seed products.

SOY MILK. It's a shock after you're used to cow's milk, but it won't cause lactose intolerance. If you can't get used to the taste, try using it in recipes and products such as pudding where adding milk is required.

YOGURT. Research shows that yogurt with active cultures may be a good source of calcium for many people with lactose intolerance, even though it is fairly high in lactose. According to the National Digestive Diseases Information Clearinghouse, evidence shows that the bacterial cultures used in making yogurt produce some of the lactase enzyme required for proper digestion.

JUST PLAIN YOGURT

Originally produced as a way to preserve milk, yogurt is one of the most digestive tract-friendly foods you can eat, and its intestinal benefits have been recorded since the 16th century. The following yogurt facts pertain to regular yogurt with live cultures, not to yogurt products such as frozen treats.

- One cup a day can reduce total cholesterol by more than three percent.
- It fights the harmful bacteria responsible for diarrhea. Studies indicate that those who eat only yogurt during a severe bout may recover twice as quickly as those who are treated medically or by other means.
- It has a similar effect on the colon as fiber and can be used to maintain bowel regularity or relieve constipation.
- It's a good source of calcium and can be used in place of milk by those who are lactose intolerant because the bacteria in yogurt produce lactase.
- It helps relieve the symptoms of irritable bowel syndrome.
- A 1 ¾ cup serving has the same amount of calcium as about 4 cups milk.

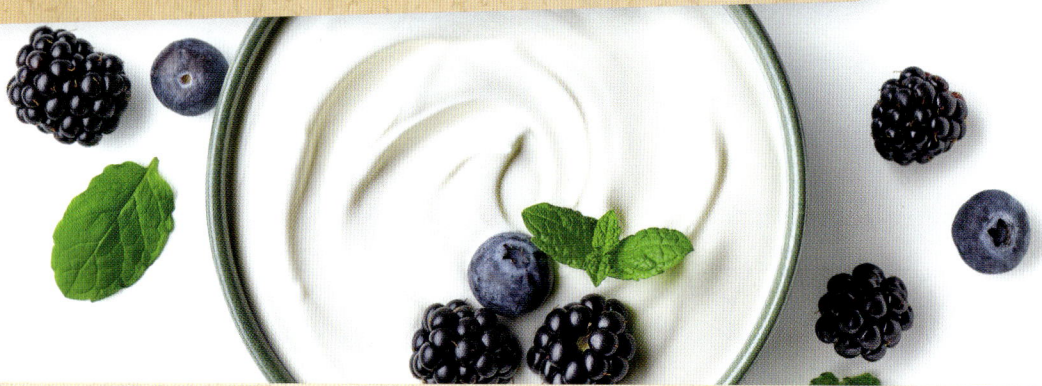

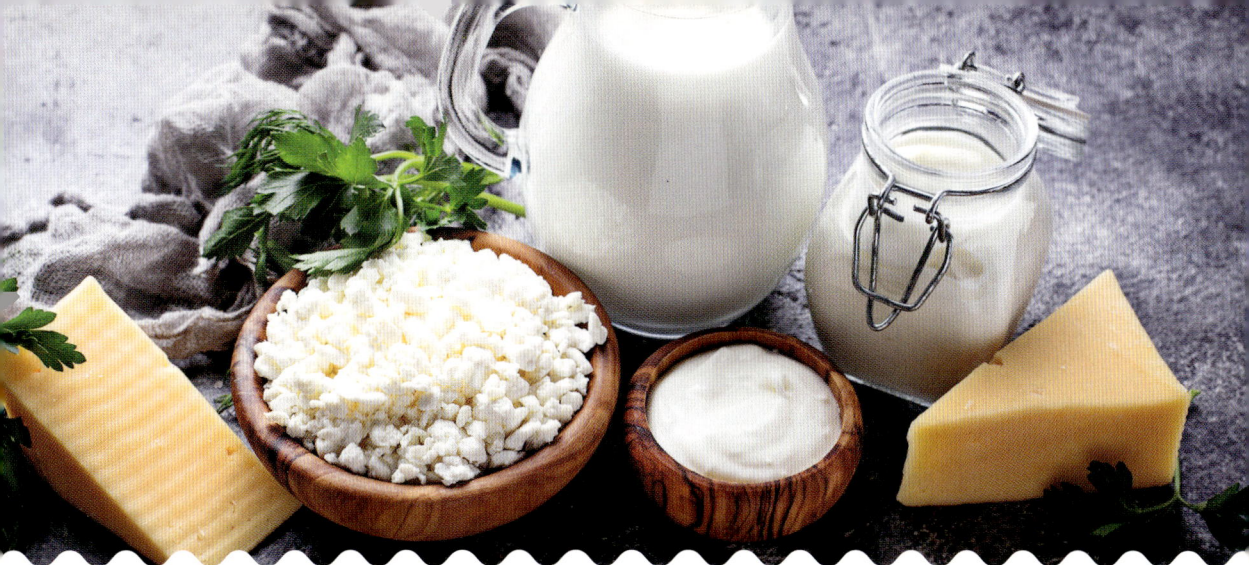

TOOLS FROM THE DRAWER

MAGNIFYING GLASS. Check the product content listed on the label for hidden milk. The print may be tiny, but looking for milk could save you from misery. These are the buzzwords to look for: whey, curds, milk by-products, dry milk solids, nonfat dry milk, milk powder, milk sugar, casein, galactose, skim whey protein concentrate.

MEASURING CUP. Most people who suffer lactose intolerance do produce an amount of lactase. So, if that 8-ounce glass of milk you drink in the morning backfires, divide it up. Measure out ⅓ cup three times a day and see if you can handle the smaller amount.

NOTEBOOK. Keep a food diary. First, cut out *all* milk products for 3 to 4 weeks. Then, add back small amounts of milk at a meal, ¼ to ½ cup at a time, and see what you can tolerate. Gradually increase or decrease the amount according to your symptoms.

UNMASKING THE MILK

These all may contain milk that you're not aware of:

- Bread
- Cereals
- Pancakes
- Chocolate
- Soups, especially cream-based
- Pudding
- Salad dressing
- Sherbet
- Instant cocoa mix
- Soft candy
- Frozen dinners
- Cookie mix
- Hot dogs

The amounts may be negligible, but if you're very sensitive to lactose, even the tiny amounts of milk can cause symptoms.

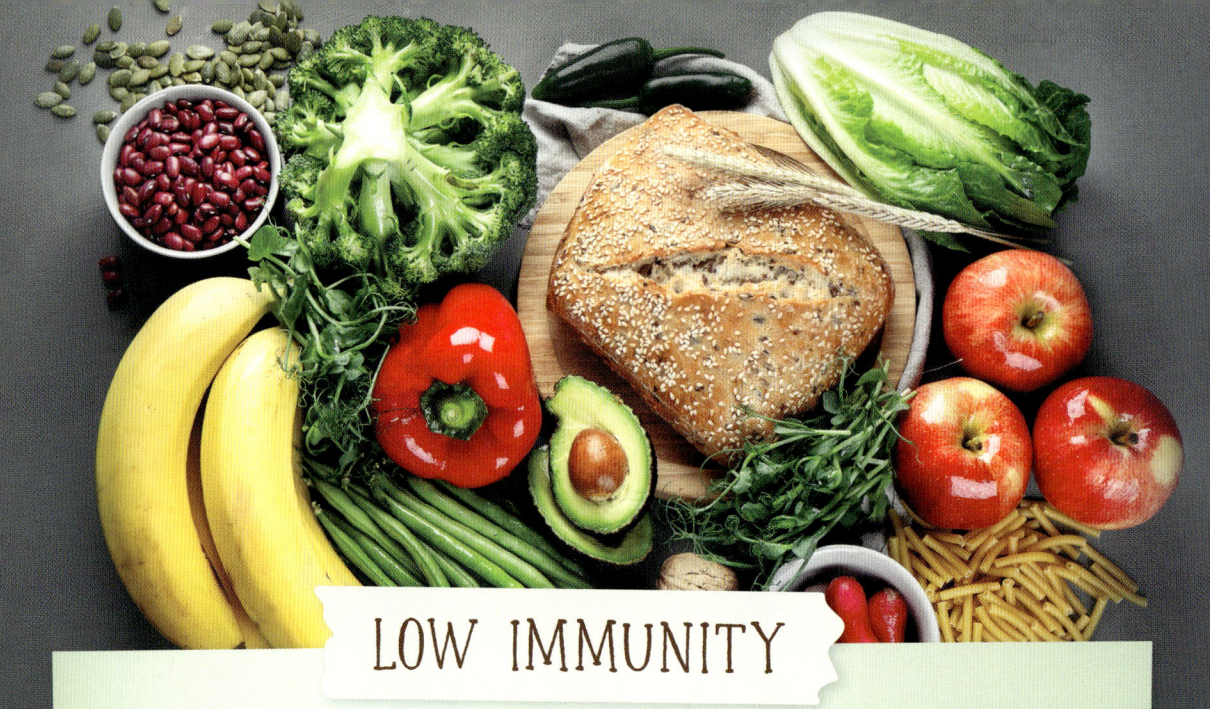

LOW IMMUNITY

In medical terms, having immunity means that you have resistance to infection or a specified disease. So if you have low immunity, it means your immune system isn't up to par and that you have a greater chance of getting the germ-du-jour. There are many factors that affect your body's response to a foreign invader, including how you're feeling at the moment you're introduced to a suspect germ. But if you consistently end up with the latest flu bug or stomach virus, your immune system may be running on empty.

WHEN THE ENEMY STRIKES

When something enters your body that is viewed by the immune system as harmful, your body goes into a state of heightened alert. When your immune system is healthy and all systems are go, these foreign invaders, or antigens, are typically met by a barrage of antibodies, which are produced by white blood cells. These antibodies latch on to antigens and set into action all the events that lead to the invader's eventual demise.

If things in your immune system are not working properly, you become less able to fight off those foreign invaders. Eventually they set up shop in your body and you get sick. An impaired immune system can make you more susceptible to colds and other merely frustrating illnesses, but it can also make you more at risk for developing cancer.

Science is proving that getting enough of the right nutrients can help you build your immune system. Scientific studies are discovering that avoiding something as simple as a cold or something as life threatening as cancer may all be affected by what you stock in your kitchen.

KITCHEN CURES

ALMONDS. Eat a handful of almonds for your daily dose of vitamin E. An immune-strengthening antioxidant, studies have found that vitamin E deficiency causes major problems in the integrity of the immune system.

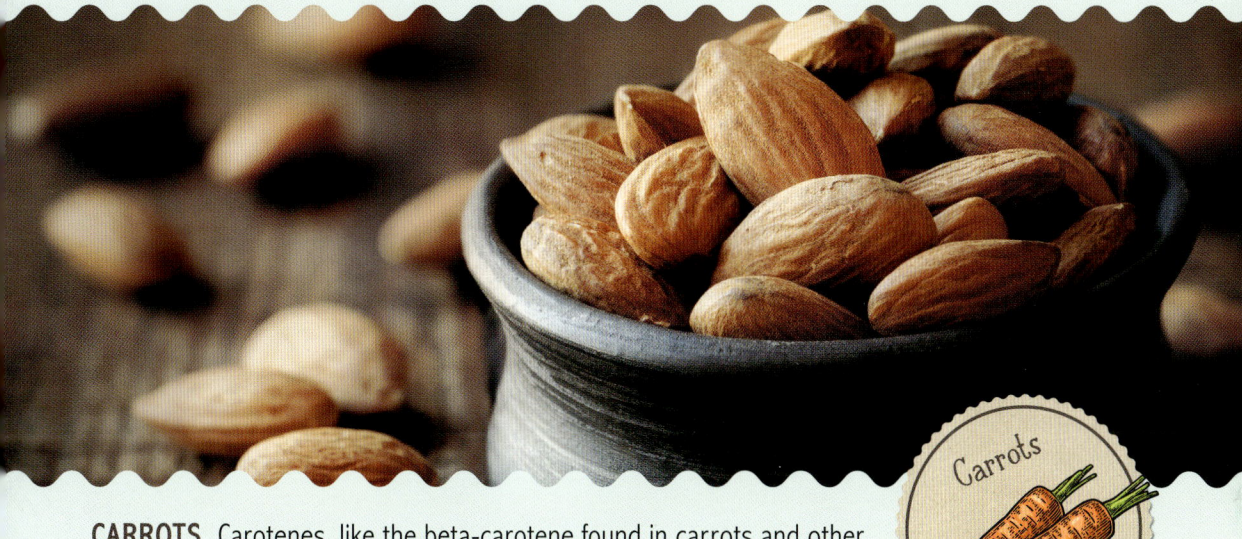

CARROTS. Carotenes, like the beta-carotene found in carrots and other red, yellow, orange, and dark-green leafy vegetables, are the protectors of the immune system, specifically the thymus gland. Carotenes strengthen white blood cell production, and numerous studies have shown that eating foods rich in beta-carotene helps the body fight off infection more easily.

CHICKEN. Selenium is a trace mineral that is vital to the development and movement of white blood cells in the body. A 3-ounce piece of chicken will give you almost half your daily needs.

CRAB. A zinc deficiency can zap your immune system. Zinc acts as a catalyst in the immune system's killer response to foreign bodies, and it protects the body from damage from invading cells. It also is a necessary ingredient for white blood cell function. Nosh on 3 ounces fresh or canned crab and you've got one-third of your recommended daily allowance (RDA) of this immune-enhancing nutrient.

GARLIC. Garlic is well-known for its antibacterial and antiviral properties. It's even been thought to help prevent cancer. Researchers think these benefits stem from garlic's amazing effect on the immune system. One study found that people who ate more garlic had more of the natural killer white blood cells than those who didn't eat garlic.

GUAVA. Go a little tropical with this tasty fruit and get more than twice your daily vitamin C needs. Vitamin C acts as an immune enhancer by helping white blood cells perform at their peak and quickening the response time of the immune system.

KALE. A cup of kale will give you your daily requirement of vitamin A. Vitamin A is an antioxidant that helps your body fight cancer cells and is essential in the formation of white blood cells. Vitamin A also increases the ability of antibodies to respond to invaders.

NAVY BEANS. Everybody needs a little folic acid (it's the most common nutrient deficiency in the United States). And not getting enough of this vital nutrient can actually shrink vital immune system fighters like your thymus and lymph nodes. To make sure you're getting your fill of folic acid, try popping open a can of navy beans with dinner. One cup gets you half of your recommended daily allowance (RDA) of folic acid.

PORK. Not getting enough vitamin B6 can keep your immune system from functioning at its best. Eating 3 ounces of lean roast pork will provide you with one-third of most adults' daily requirements for this immune-helping vitamin.

SHIITAKE MUSHROOMS. Throw a few shiitake mushrooms in your stir-fry and you may prevent your yearly cold. Scientists have discovered that specific components of shiitake mushrooms boost your immune system and act as antiviral agents.

YOGURT. Yogurt seems to have a marked effect on the immune system. It strengthens white blood cells and helps the immune system produce antibodies. One study found that people who ate 6 ounces of yogurt a day avoided colds, hay fever, and diarrhea. Another study found that yogurt could be an ally in the body's war against cancer.

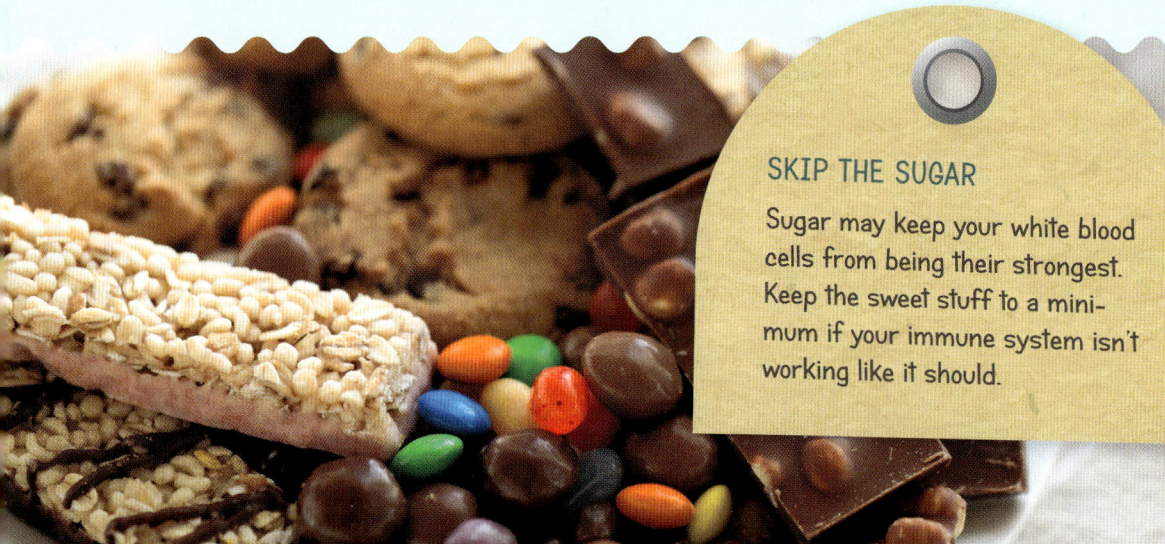

SKIP THE SUGAR

Sugar may keep your white blood cells from being their strongest. Keep the sweet stuff to a minimum if your immune system isn't working like it should.

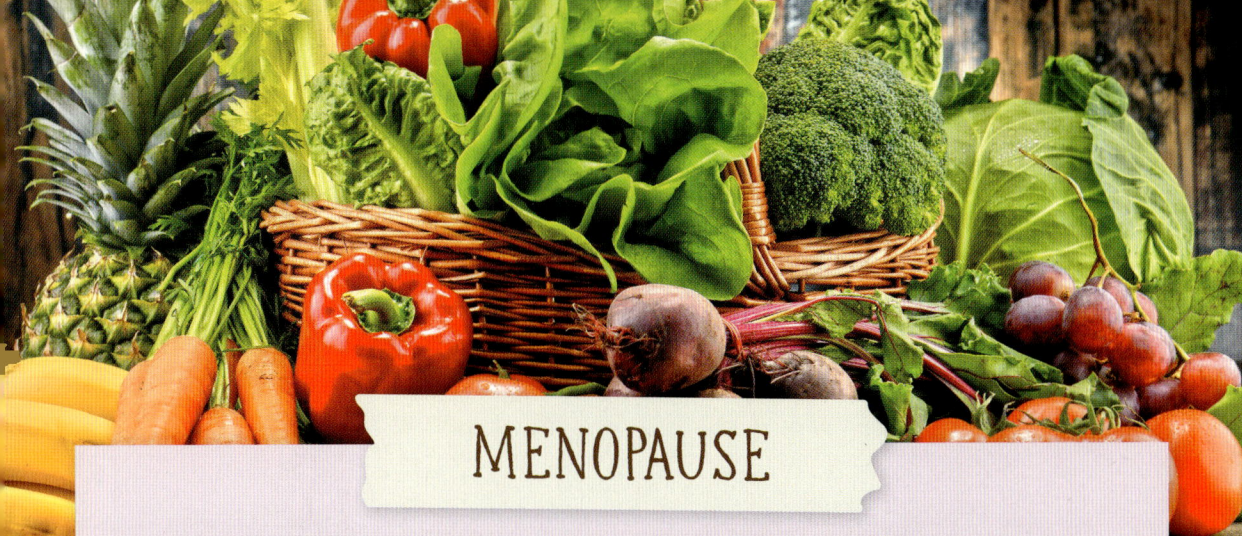

MENOPAUSE

Most women look forward to the cessation of menstruation and all its associated annoyances. It happens to every woman sometime between the ages of 40 and 60, and on average at age 51. But menopause isn't just your last period. It's a process of bodily changes and a reduction in female hormones, and it occurs over several years.

These are some of the pre-menopausal changes:

- Estrogen levels begin to drop off around age 30.
- Egg production and release slow down, usually during the 40s.
- Menstrual cycles change. They become longer or shorter, lighter or heavier. Months—or only a week or two—may elapse between periods.
- Whatever happens this time will change next time.

Overall, it takes an average of about four years to get through these changes and cross that menopause threshold, but once menstruation has been absent for a full year, you are pronounced "postmenopausal."

In the meantime, as menopause is galloping to the finishing line, it's dragging along a lot of unpleasant symptoms: hot flashes, vaginal dryness, bladder infection, incontinence, heart palpitations, achy joints, dry or itchy skin, headache, insomnia, weight gain, thinning hair, increased facial hair, mood swings, memory problems, and change in sexual drive.

Obviously, this transition requires some medical guidance, since the consequences can be much more serious than the profuse sweating of a hot flash. But there are ways to curb some of the menopausal symptoms right in your own kitchen. And since menopause is nothing to cure, but rather to endure, curbing those problems so simply can be a big relief.

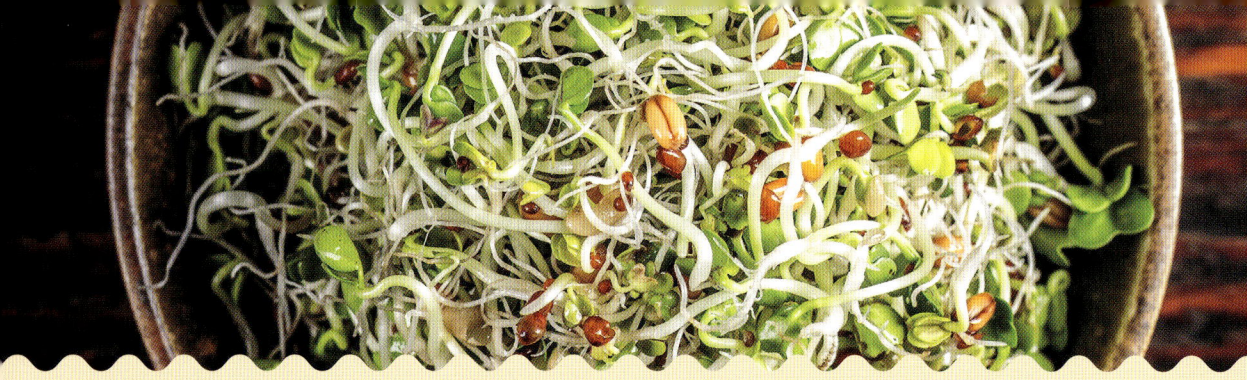

KITCHEN CURES

ALFALFA SPROUTS. Their plant estrogen may help prevent thinning of the vaginal walls. Sprinkle on a salad or use in a stir-fry. Make sure your sprouts are clean before you eat them, though. Raw sprouts can be contaminated with the *E. coli* bacteria. Flaxseed is rich in natural estrogen, too.

LIME JUICE. Mix 5 to 10 drops with 1 teaspoon organic sugar and 1 cup pomegranate juice. Drink two to three times a day to relieve hot flashes.

ORANGES. The vitamin C in oranges is a natural immune booster. It also guards your skin against damage. Other C-rich foods include grapefruits, berries, papayas, green leafy veggies, peppers, and sweet potatoes.

PARSLEY. Joint aches and pains are a common complaint of menopause and parsley tea may bring relief. Steep a spoonful in a cup of boiling water for ten minutes, sweeten to taste, and drink two to three times a day. If you can stand the strong taste, add more parsley.

SAGE. This has estrogenlike properties and can help reduce sweating and hot flashes. Steep 1 to 2 fresh leaves or a spoonful of dried sage in 1 cup boiling water for ten minutes. Sweeten with honey, add lemon if desired. Drink a cup or two every day. Or, use sage as a spice on vegetables or to season meats.

SARDINES. Canned sardines, with bones and oil, are rich in bone-building calcium. Because loss of bone density is a common companion to menopause and can lead to osteoporosis, calcium-rich foods are important. Low fat dairy foods, sesame seeds, nuts, and legumes also should be added to your diet.

SOY. It comes in many forms and they're all great at relieving symptoms such as hot flashes and vaginal dryness, preventing loss of bone density, and lowering cholesterol. Try adding tofu, soy milk, and tempeh to your diet.

MENSTRUAL PROBLEMS

Menstruation is the simple process of shedding the old uterine lining to make way for a new one. In other words, it's the body's way of sweeping out the cobwebs at the end of the month in preparation for the arrival of a new egg and a new cycle; all a part of the natural baby-making process with one goal in mind: conception.

Most women will experience in the neighborhood of 400 menstrual cycles in their childbearing lifetime. And that's a lot of cycles that can cause problems: bloat, backache, leg aches, headaches, acne, cramps, and mood swings. Serious menstrual problems require medical treatment, since many can lead to infertility, infection, and in some cases, death. But some of the milder problems can be relieved with simple kitchen cures. And any menstrual relief, no matter how slight, is welcome!

KITCHEN CURES

BASIL. This can relieve some of the normal pain associated with menstruation because it contains caffeic acid, which has an analgesic, or pain-killing, effect. Thyme is also high in caffeic acid. Use it as a spice in cooking meat and vegetables or Italian dishes. Or steep the herb into tea, adding 2 tablespoons thyme or basil leaves to 1 pint boiling water. Cover tightly and let cool to room temperature. Drink ½ to 1 cup an hour for painful menstruation.

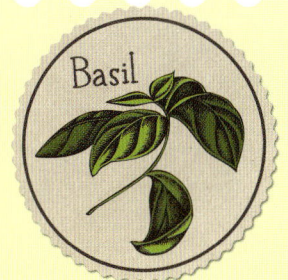

BUCKWHEAT. It's high in bioflavonoids and can reduce heavy bleeding when taken with vitamin C. Try it in buckwheat pancakes. Fruits, nuts, and seeds are high in bioflavonoids, too.

CINNAMON. This has anti-inflammatory and antispasmodic properties that relieve cramps. Use as a tea, or sprinkle on toast or sweet rolls. If you have a heavy period, drinking cinnamon tea the day before or during your period may help.

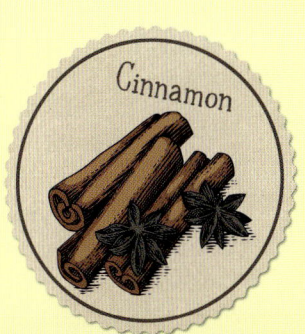

CITRUS FRUITS. Eat or drink with your meals to enhance iron absorption into the body, since iron is easily depleted during menstruation.

DRIED APRICOTS. These are high in iron, which is important during menstruation because iron supplies can be depleted with heavy bleeding. Other iron-rich foods are: liver, legumes, shellfish, and fortified breads and cereals.

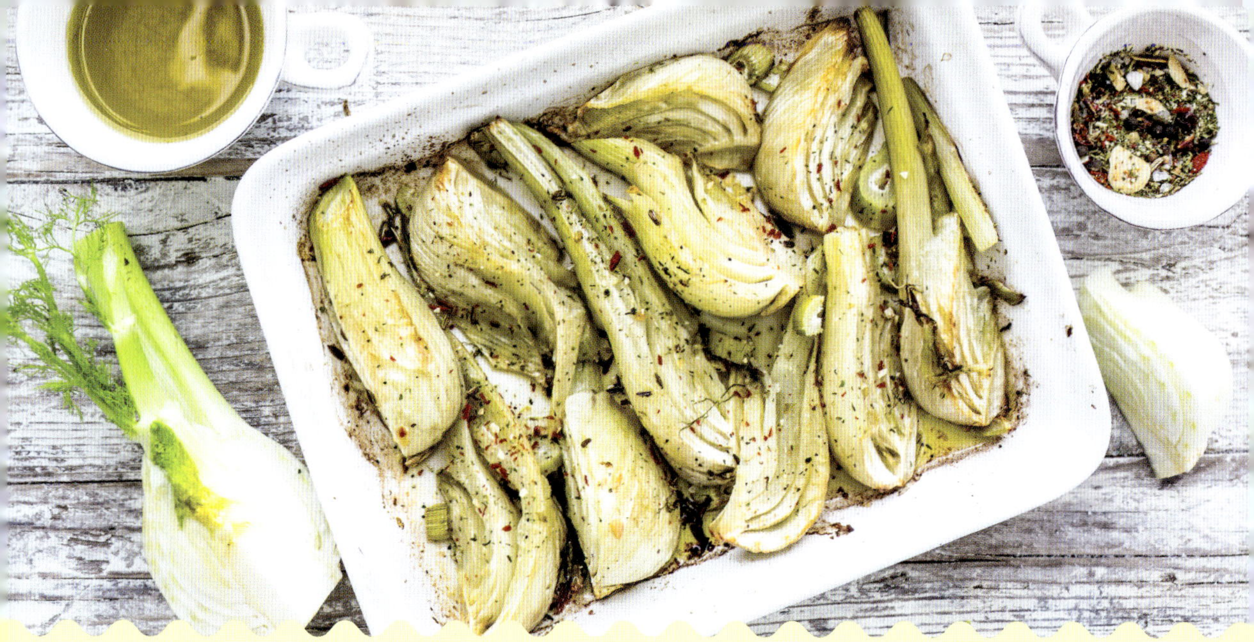

FENNEL. Another cramp cure, this spice promotes better circulation to the ovaries. Crush 1 teaspoon fennel seeds into a powder. Add to 1 cup boiling water, steep five minutes, strain, and drink hot.

GINGER. This is a cramp reliever, and as an added bonus it sometimes can make irregular periods regular. Use in cookies, cake, and candy or as a spice in vegetables and stir-fries. Tea may be the most effective form, however: put ½ teaspoon in 1 cup boiling water, and drink three times a day.

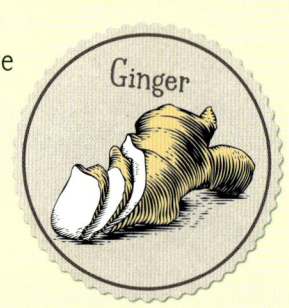

HOT WATER. Put it in a hot water bottle and place on the abdomen to relieve cramps. Or, soak a kitchen towel, then wring out excess water, heat in microwave for a minute, and place on abdomen. Be careful not to burn yourself, however.

MINT. Either peppermint or wintergreen can relieve cramps. Steep into a tea and drink a cup or two a day. Try sucking on mint candy, too.

MUSTARD. A tablespoon or two of powdered mustard in a basin of nice warm water can relieve cramps, but don't drink it. Soak your feet in it to reap the relaxing effects.

RED MEAT. It's loaded with iron as well as zinc, which can be depleted during menses, too. Zinc is necessary for healthy bones, and a zinc deficiency may result in amenorrhea. Other iron- and zinc-rich foods: poultry, fish, green leafy vegetables.

WATER. Drink plenty of it. Dehydration can cause the body to produce a hormone called vasopressin that contributes to cramps.

HERBAL CURES

Typically, the cure for female complaints has been one or more herbs. Some of the more common are found in most spice racks, but here are a few you might wish to seek out to stock that menstrual medicinal herb rack.

CHAMOMILE. This is known to be a reliable cramp reliever. Place ½ ounce in a 1-pint jar and cover with boiling water. Steep for one hour, strain, and drink a cup every hour or two. Use honey to sweeten to taste. This is a particularly relaxing tea just before bed.

LEMON BALM. This is another cramp reliever, also used for menstruation delayed by stress and tension. Lemon balm also has a mild sedative effect. Make the tea by placing 1 ounce of the herb in 1 quart boiling water, then letting it cool to room temperature. Strain and drink ½ cup per hour until the cramps are gone.

RASPBERRY LEAF. Place 1 ounce raspberry leaf in 1 pint water, then bring to a slow boil. Cover and simmer on the lowest heat 30 to 40 minutes. Cool, stir, strain, bottle. Sweeten to taste. One raspberry leaf contains: 408 mg calcium, 446 mg potassium, 106 mg magnesium, 4 mg manganese, and 3.3 mg iron.

YARROW. A tea made with this herb can stop excessive or prolonged bleeding. It can be taken during the period for bleeding relief or at the beginning to make the entire period easier.

MOTION SICKNESS

It can happen almost anywhere—in the backseat of your family van, on the Tilt-a-Whirl at the county fair, on the bumpy airplane ride to grandma's. Anything that moves has the potential to give you a green hue and leave you wishing the world would put on the brakes. Thankfully, most people only deal with motion sickness on occasion. And following some simple tips can help avert those rare bouts.

TUMMY TURBULENCE

So why does your tummy do cartwheels every time you sail, fly, or ride? Motion sickness is purely a matter of miscommunication. When you're cruising down the road focused on a book or a person, your eyes tell your brain that you're not moving, but your inner ear tells the brain a different story. For instance, you and your girlfriends are going for a long-awaited women-only weekend. All six of you pile in your friend's minivan. You pop in the passenger seat and as soon as you get on the road, you're turned around chatting with your buddies. You see only your stationary friends sitting in the back of the van, so your eyes tell your brain that you're sitting in a room catching up with old pals. But the fluid in your inner ear is sloshing around with every bump and turn. Your brain is getting mixed signals. And in the confusion, your brain triggers your tummy and you start feeling sick. Next thing you know, you and the girls are forced to make a pit stop.

SYMPTOMS OF A SPINNING HEAD

No one can completely avoid motion sickness. Even astronauts have bouts of nausea every now and then. For most people, motion sickness comes on fairly quickly and usually involves one of these symptoms: sweating, hyperventilation, dizziness, paleness, sensation of spinning, loss of appetite, and of course, nausea.

KITCHEN CURES

APPLE JUICE. Drink a glass of apple juice with your pre-travel low fat meal. Giving your body a bit of sugar with fluids before you start your journey should help you down the road. And if you start feeling ill, sipping (not gulping) some juice may help you feel better. Almost any non-citrus juice will do. Citrus juice irritates an already unstable stomach.

CRACKERS. Take these easily digestible snacks along and nibble on them every couple of hours to help prevent nausea and vomiting. An empty stomach makes it more likely that you will get sick.

GINGER. Ginger has long been known as an herbal remedy for queasiness, but modern science has proved this spice has merit, especially for motion sickness. One study discovered that ginger was actually better than over-the-counter motion sickness drugs. Make a ginger tea to take along with you when you're traveling by cutting 10 to 12 slices of fresh ginger and placing them in a pot with 1 quart water. Boil for ten minutes. Strain out the ginger, and add ½ cup honey or maple syrup for sweetening if you like.

LOW FAT FOODS. If you eat a low fat meal before you head out on your trip, you may avoid getting sick. Eating something before you leave makes your stomach more capable of handling the ups and downs of the road. Experts say not eating destabilizes the stomach's electrical signals, making you susceptible to nausea and vomiting.

PEPPERMINT CANDIES OR LOZENGES. If you start feeling sick, get out the peppermints. Not only will you end up with fresh minty breath when you arrive at your destination, you'll also calm your queasiness. And if you're traveling with little ones, try placing 1 drop peppermint oil on their tongues before the trip. It may quash the queasy feeling.

TEA. Sip on some warm tea if you start feeling sick. Warm beverages tend to be easier on a nauseated tummy than a tall glass of cold water. Go for the decaf brew; caffeinated drinks aren't a good idea for unstable stomachs.

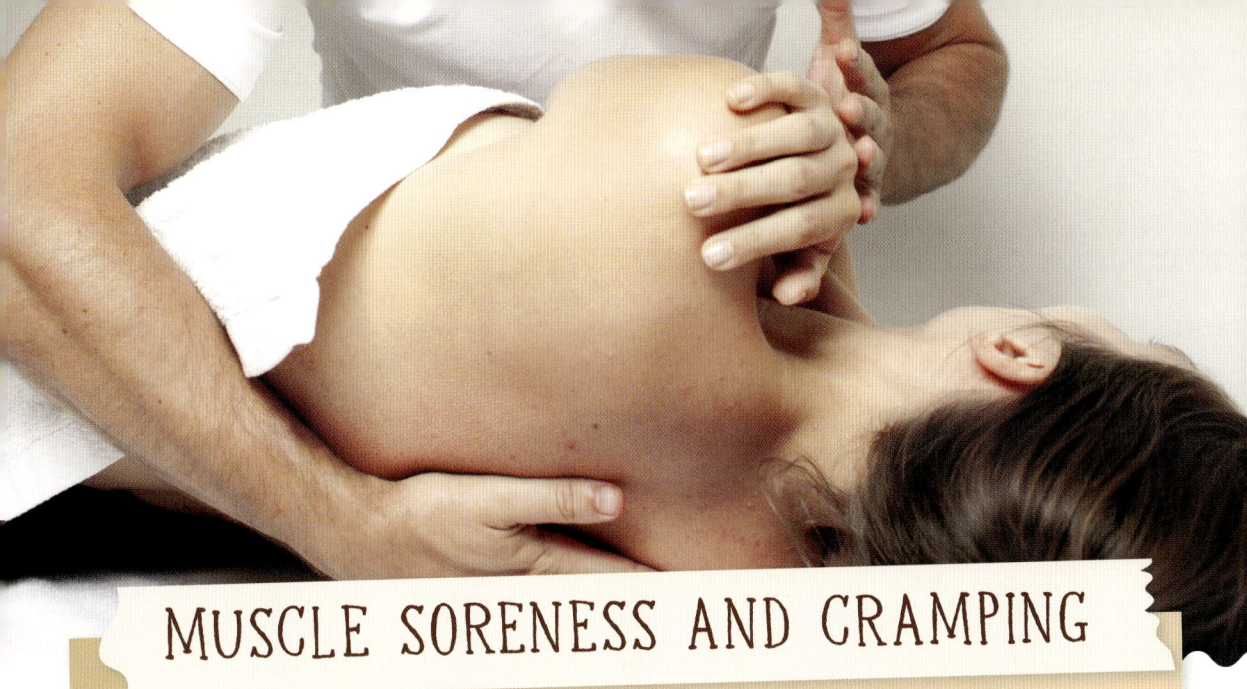

MUSCLE SORENESS AND CRAMPING

You've made your New Year's resolution: You are going to get in shape. So you venture into your local health club and decide to try the low/high aerobics class for people who have been out of circulation for a while. By the time you get home, though, your muscles have gone on strike. The next day you can barely muster enough strength to make it out of bed, and you spend the day walking like you've been riding the range a bit too long. You'll take it slower next time. But what can you do right now to ease the pain?

MUSCLE MAYHEM

The vast array of muscles in your body is what allows you to do something as simple as picking up a fork or as complicated as a kickboxing routine. Muscles are a complex weave of fibers that work with your brain and skeletal system to give you the agility to return that volley across the tennis court. When you're taking care to stretch and strengthen your muscles, they are your greatest ally. But when they don't work like they should or they get injured, you have a very painful problem on your hands.

Strains are one of the most common reasons for aching muscles. When you strain a muscle, it means you've worked it too hard, causing the muscle fibers to pull and tear. If you haven't worked out for a while and then head back full throttle without preparing your muscles for the trauma they're about to experience, or if you're an experienced exerciser and you don't warm up properly, you risk getting a strained muscle. At best, a strained muscle will leave you sore for a few days; at worst, you could end up with a "pulled" muscle, one whose fibers have been totally torn.

Another common muscle malady is cramps, or spasms. Muscle cramps happen when the muscle isn't getting enough blood, and in response to the restricted blood flow the muscle shortens and tightens. The slowdown in blood flow can be caused by a variety of problems:

- A deficiency in essential nutrients for maximum muscle power, such as sodium, calcium, and potassium
- Depletion of the muscles' energy supply of glycogen
- Overworked muscles
- Holding the same position for too long

Whatever the reason, when blood doesn't reach your muscles the way it should, your muscles can turn into balls of pain.

Your first priority is to give your muscles some rest and take a few ideas from the kitchen that will help you feel better, fast.

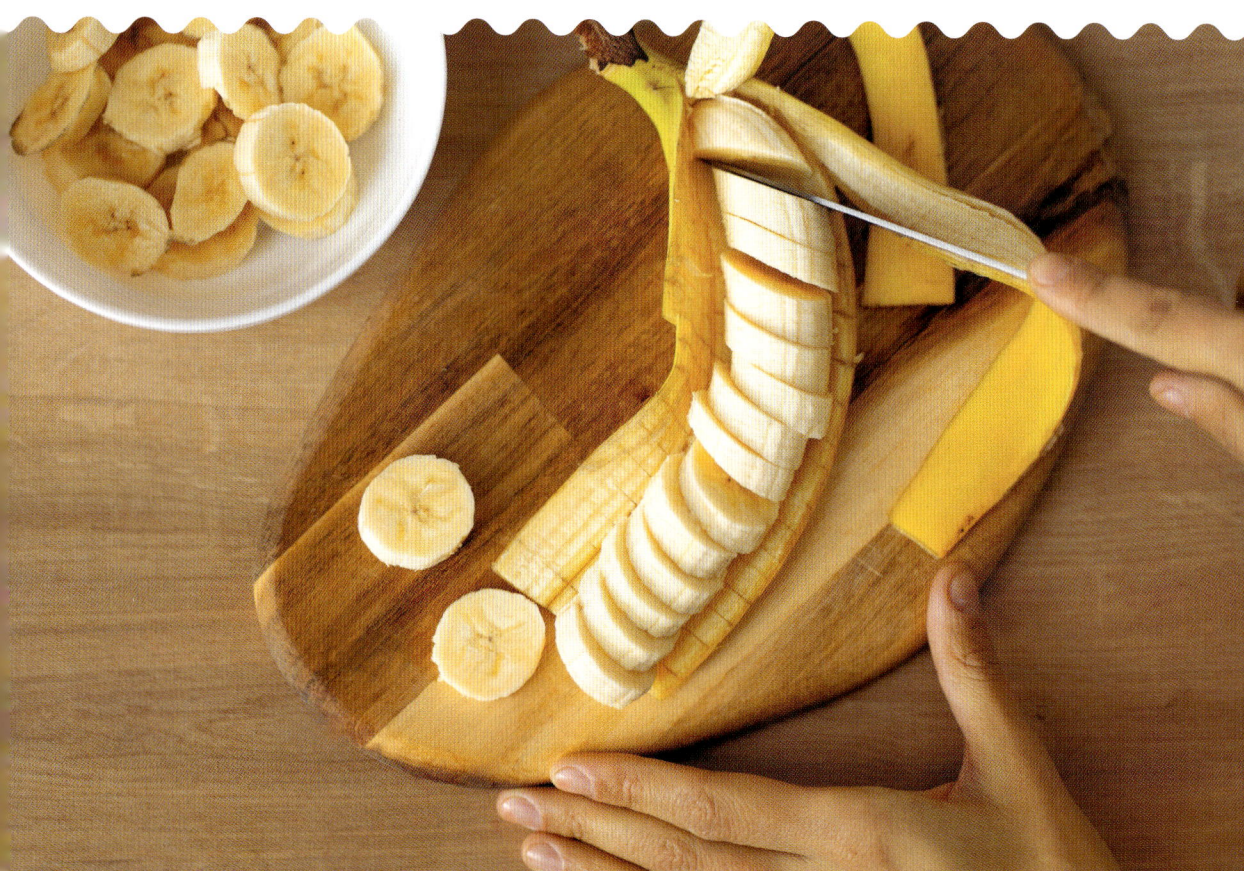

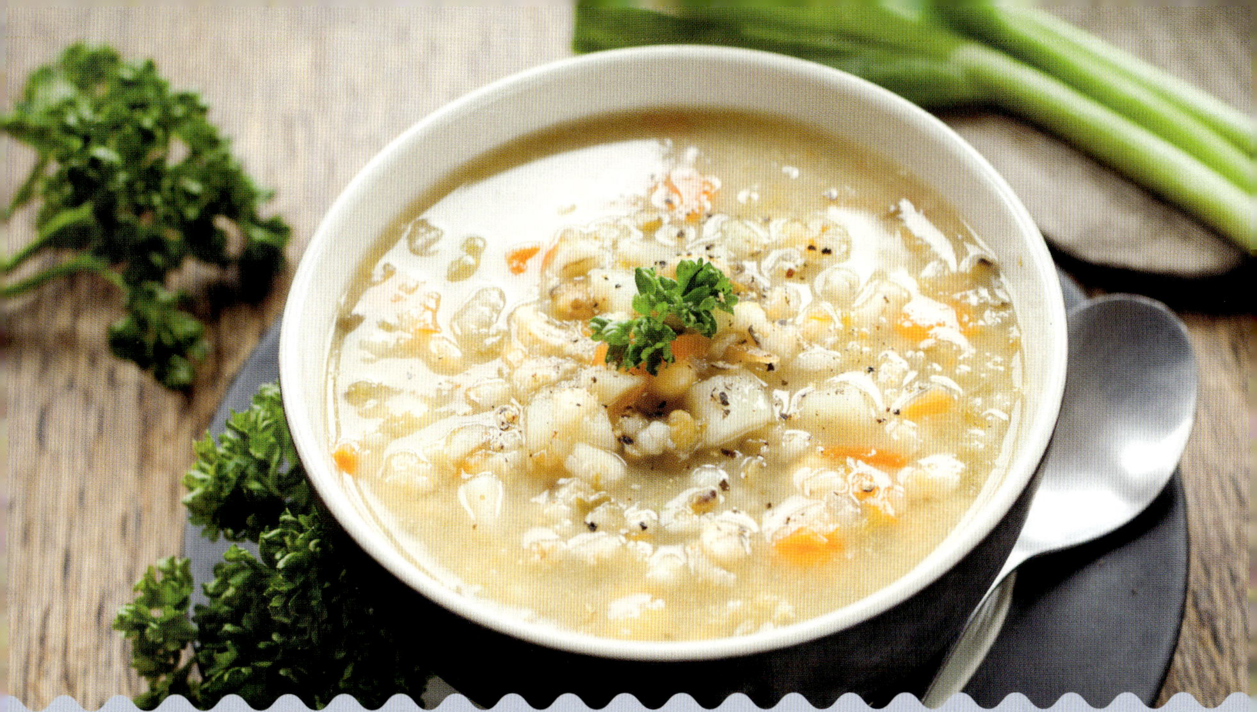

KITCHEN CURES

BANANA. Eat a banana or two a day and you may cut down your cramping. That's because a potassium deficiency may be to blame for muscle cramps. One banana has 450 mg of the muscle-protecting nutrient.

BOUILLON. Sipping some warm soup before heading out for a long bike ride may not sound appealing, but it may help you skip the muscle cramps. Drink 1 cup beef or chicken bouillon before you ride. It helps you replace the sodium you lose when you sweat.

MILK. Getting adequate amounts of calcium in your diet may help curtail your cramps. Women especially seem to need plenty of calcium for muscle health. Three glasses of milk a day will meet the calcium needs of most adults.

ROSEMARY. A few leaves of rosemary can help reduce swelling in strained muscles. Use either fresh or dried leaves; fresh has more of the volatile oils. The herb has four anti-inflammatory properties, which can help calm inflamed muscle tissue and speed healing. Because rosemary is easily absorbed through the skin, placing a cloth soaked with a rosemary wash will help ease the pain. Here's how to make a rosemary wash: Put 1 ounce rosemary leaves in a 1-pint jar and fill the jar with boiling water. Cover and let stand for 30 minutes. Apply the wash to the area two or three times a day.

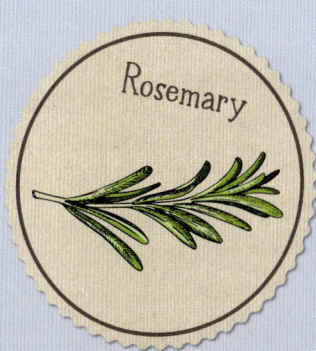
Rosemary

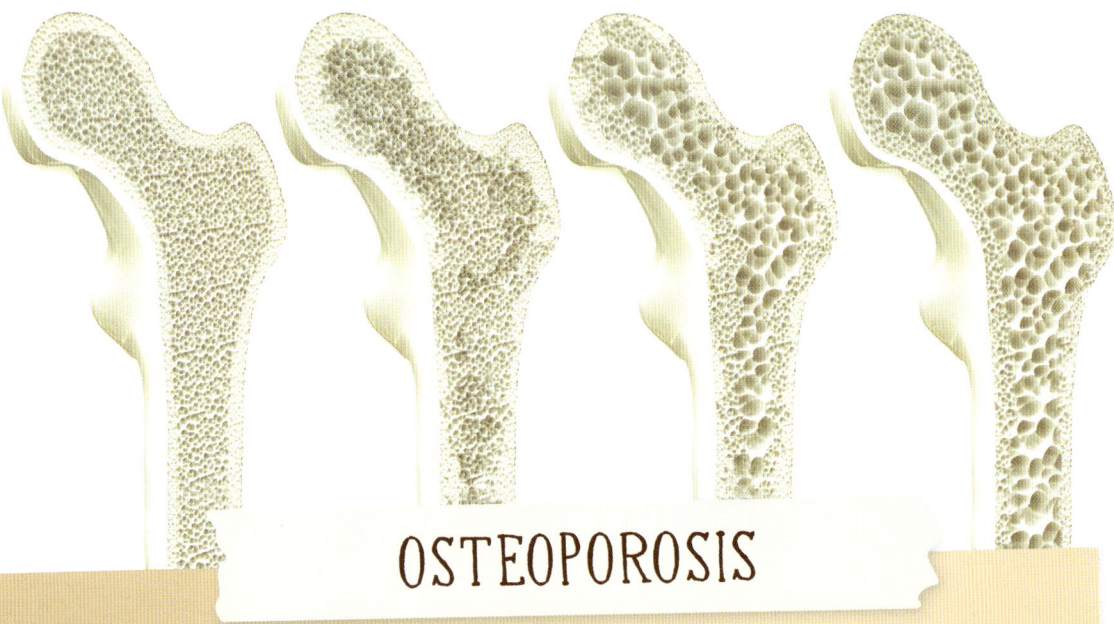

OSTEOPOROSIS

Though most people associate osteoporosis with older people, the disease strikes young and old alike. But osteoporosis does become much more common as you age—affecting one in two women over age 50.

As you grow your bones get stronger and longer. By the time you reach the age of 20, you've got 98 percent of your bone mass; by the time you reach your thirtieth birthday, your bones are their strongest. If you were able to take a look inside your bones during those peak years, you'd see a hard outer shell and something that looks like a honeycomb on the inside. About 80 percent of your bone mass is that tough, hard outer bone called cortical bone. The rest of your bone make-up is the honeycomblike material called trabecular bone. After you hit 30, your bone mass begins to decline. Trabecular bone is typically the first to lose critical density, and as you get older, cortical bone mass also declines, but at a slower pace.

Osteoporosis literally means porous bones. That means someone diagnosed with the disease has lost so much density that there's not much there to hold their bones together, putting them at greater risk for bone breaks and fractures. The National Osteoporosis Foundation calls osteoporosis the "silent disease" because there are virtually no symptoms of bone loss. Unless you're aware of the risk factors and take action, you may not know you have the disease until some benign bump on the garage door turns into a fracture.

WHO GETS OSTEOPOROSIS?

Being Caucasian or Asian, female, small-framed, and underweight are major risk factors for thinning bones. And so is being postmenopausal. That's because estrogen is vital to bone strength, keeping bones strong by stimulating bone-building substances called osteoblasts and suppressing bone-destroying substances called osteoclasts. Estrogen also helps the body absorb and use calcium more efficiently. As women approach menopause, estrogen production steadily declines and the protection it provides against osteoporosis is lost. But one of the greatest risk factors for osteoporosis is something you can't see and you can't control—heredity. Other risk factors include: not getting enough calcium, having an eating disorder, using certain medications such as corticosteroids, not exercising, and smoking.

Thankfully, there are many ways you can combat and even reverse the damaging effects of this bone-thinning disease, and the earlier you start the better. Why not try some of the bone boosters in your kitchen?

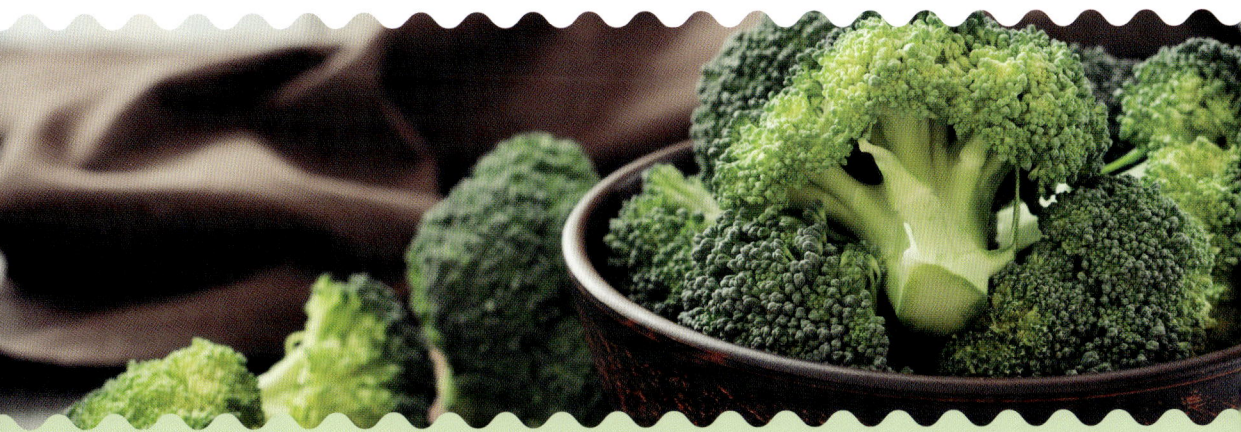

KITCHEN CURES

APPLES. Boron is a trace mineral that helps your body hold on to calcium—the building block of bones. It even acts as a mild estrogen replacement, and losing estrogen is instrumental in speeding bone loss. Boron is found in apples and other fruits such as pears, grapes, dates, raisins, and peaches. It's also in nuts such as almonds, peanuts, and hazelnuts.

BANANA. Eat a banana a day to build your bones. Studies have found that women who have diets high in potassium also have stronger bones in their spines and hips. Researchers think this is related to potassium's ability to keep blood healthy and balanced so the body doesn't have to suck calcium from the skeleton to keep blood up to par.

BROCCOLI. Eat ½ cup broccoli to get your daily dose of vitamin K. Studies are finding that postmenopausal women with low levels of this vital vitamin are more likely to have osteoporosis.

MARGARINE. Slather a teaspoon of low trans fatty margarine on your toast for a dose of vitamin D. Vitamin D helps the body absorb calcium, a necessary ingredient to bone health.

MILK. When it comes to strong bones, getting enough calcium is a must. One cup of milk can provide 300 mg of the 1,000 to 1,200 mg of calcium the government recommends you get every day. But milk is not the only calcium-rich food on the market. See "Mooove Over Milk," on the next page, for more ideas on how to add this bone-strengthening mineral to your diet.

ORANGE JUICE. Grab a glass of OJ to get your vitamin C. Necessary for the body processes that rebuild bones, getting enough vitamin C is vital to preventing osteoporosis. Grab some calcium-fortified orange juice and get a healthy dose of bone-building nutrients.

PEANUT BUTTER. A recent review of studies on nutrition and osteoporosis found that magnesium was a vital component to strengthening, preserving, and rebuilding bones. You can get 50 mg of magnesium by eating 2 tablespoons of peanut butter.

PINEAPPLE JUICE. Drink a cup of pineapple juice and give your body some manganese. Studies are finding that manganese deficiency is a predictor of osteoporosis. Other manganese sources are oatmeal, nuts, beans, cereals, spinach, and tea.

MORE DO'S AND DON'TS

If you don't get enough calcium in your diet, be sure to use a supplement to help prevent osteoporosis.

- Restrict your salt. Salt may actually steal calcium away from your bones.

- Abstain from alcohol. Alcohol interferes with the way your body absorbs calcium.

- Cut the caffeine. Caffeine is a diuretic, and some experts believe drinking too much can cause your body to excrete too much calcium. Don't drink more than 2 cups of coffee or 4 cups of tea a day.

- Get some sun. To up your supply of vitamin D, be sure to catch a few rays. Spending 15 minutes a day in the sun will give you an adequate supply without causing your skin to suffer.

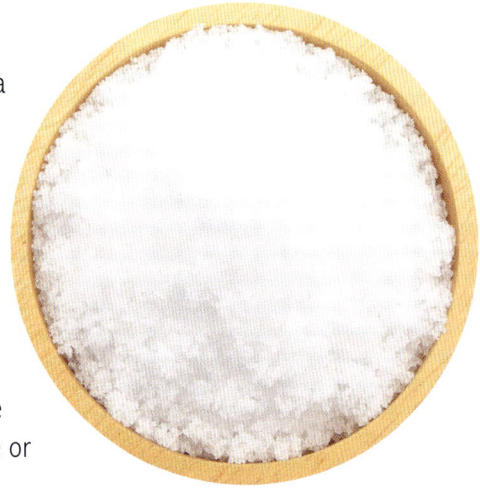

MOOOVE OVER MILK

Milk isn't the only way you can load up on calcium. There are plenty of nondairy, calcium-rich foods out there. If you're lactose intolerant or simply don't like the taste of milk but you want to be sure you're getting enough calcium, check out these calcium-rich choices.

FOOD	CALCIUM CONTENT (MILLIGRAMS)
salmon, with bones (3 ounces)	205
blackstrap molasses (1 tablespoon)	185
tofu (½ cup)	130
turnip greens (½ cup)	100
dried figs (3)	80
okra (½ cup)	50
orange (1)	45

POOR APPETITE

A poor appetite can stem from many factors. Perhaps the most common causes are emotional upset, nervousness, tension, anxiety, or depression. Stressful events, such as losing a job or a death in the family, can also make the appetite plummet. Diseases such as influenza and acute infections play a role in appetite reduction, as do anorexia nervosa and fatigue. Illegal and legal drugs, including amphetamines, antibiotics, cough and cold medications, codeine, morphine, and Demerol can take a toll on the appetite. Sometimes poor eating habits, such as continuous snacking, can lead to a poor appetite at mealtimes. A poor appetite can also be one symptom of a serious disease.

Fortunately, for minor cases of poor appetite, the kitchen is the best place to get the appetite back into gear.

Conditions 173

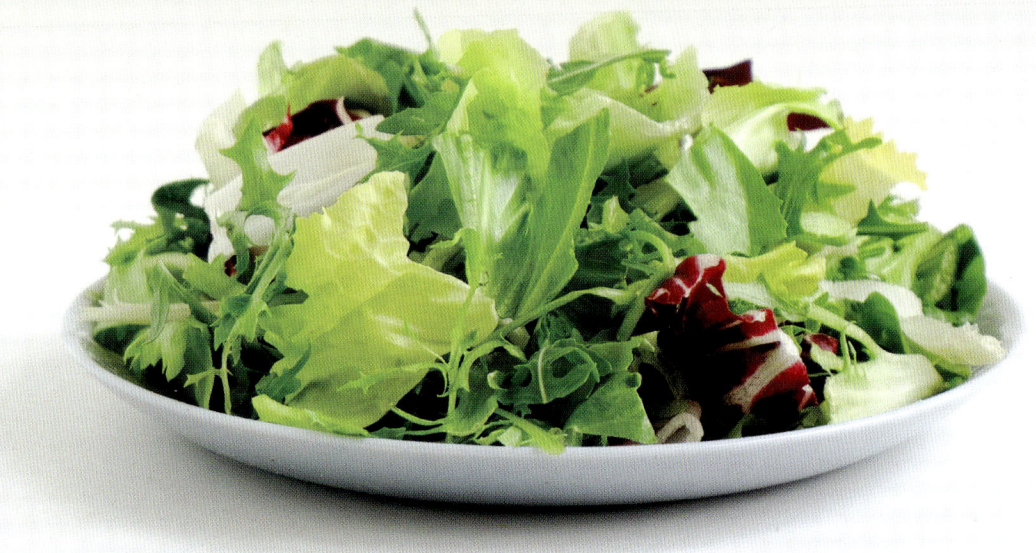

KITCHEN CURES

BITTER GREENS. Mama always told you to eat your greens. If she knew you weren't eating properly, she might add, eat your "bitter" greens. Bitter greens consist of arugula, radicchio, collards, kale, endives, escarole, mizuna, sorrel, dandelions, watercress, and red/green mustard...in other words, all those leaves you find in fancy restaurant salads. Stimulating digestion is the name of the game with bitter greens. They prompt the body into making more digestive juices and digestive enzymes. Bitter foods also stimulate the gallbladder to contract and release bile, which helps break fatty foods into small enough particles that enzymes can easily finish breaking them apart for absorption. This is important because fats carry essential fatty acids, such as heart-healthy omega-3s, along with fat-soluble vitamins A, D, E, and K and carotenoids such as beta-carotene.

CARAWAY. The early Greeks knew caraway could calm an upset stomach and used it to season foods that were hard to digest. Today unsuspecting cooks who simply love the flavor of caraway continue the tradition by adding caraway to rye bread, cabbage dishes, sauerkraut and coleslaw, pork, cheese sauces, cream soups, goose, and duck. The Germans make a caraway liqueur called Kümmel and serve it after heavy meals. One of the easiest ways to enjoy caraway is with a good helping of sauerkraut. Sauté ½ medium onion in 1 to 2 tablespoons butter. When onions turn deep golden brown, add 1 can sauerkraut and its liquid along with 1 or 2 tablespoons brown sugar and 1 teaspoon caraway seeds. Let the mixture simmer (covered) for 1 hour. Serve as a side dish with meat, poultry, or sausage.

CAYENNE PEPPER. Nothing revs up the old digestive engine like cayenne. Cayenne pepper has the power to make any dish fiery hot, but it also has a subtle flavor-enhancing quality. There is some evidence that eating hot pepper increases metabolism and the appetite. Add a few shakes of cayenne pepper to potato salad, deviled eggs, chili, and other hot dishes such as stews and soups.

FENNEL. Fennel, like its cousin caraway (both belong to the *Umbelliferae* family of herbs), is a familiar digestive aid, both for relieving stomach upset and for boosting the appetite.

GINGER. Ginger helps stimulate a tired appetite, both through its medicinal properties and its refreshing taste. Try nibbling on gingersnaps or sipping ginger ale made with real ginger. Ginger tea is also a way to start the day off on an appetizing note. To make, place ½ teaspoon powdered ginger into a cup and fill with boiling water. Cover and let stand ten minutes. Strain and sip. Don't take more than three times daily. If needed, sweeten with just a little honey.

Warning! Pregnant women should consult a doctor before taking ginger.

MINT. Peppermint refreshes the palate and revives the appetite. Make a cup of mint tea and enjoy anytime you don't feel like eating. Place 1 tablespoon mint leaves in a 1-pint jar of boiling water. Let stand 20 to 30 minutes, shaking occasionally. Strain and sip as needed. If you're tired of teas, make a glass of mint lemonade by adding a few sprigs to the lemonade mixture and letting it sit for ten minutes before sipping.

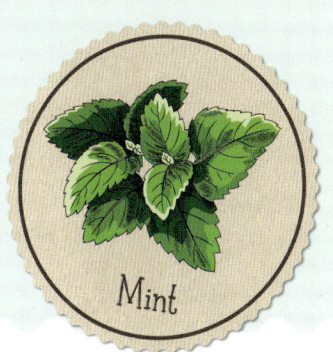
Mint

LOOK TO THE LAWN FOR HELP

Dandelions help stimulate digestion, thanks to a bitter substance called taraxacin that promotes the flow of bile from the liver and hydrochloric acid secretions from the stomach. Dandelion also helps the body to absorb nutrients and eliminate wastes more efficiently. Don't use dandelions from any lawns that may have been sprayed with chemicals or fertilizers. Dandelions are also available in some groceries and fruit and vegetable markets. Here is a recipe to get you started:

SAUTÉED DANDELIONS

Add young dandelions to your favorite stir-fry. Or sauté them with mushrooms, onions, and shredded kale and cabbage in some sesame oil. The greens cook quickly, even on low heat, so take care not to overcook. (They'll be mushy and distasteful if you do.) Remove from heat, add a dash of sesame oil and balsamic vinegar, and garnish with sesame seeds. Serve as a side dish or over rice.

Warning! Avoid dandelions if you have too much stomach acid, ulcers, diarrhea, irritable bowel syndrome, or ulcerative colitis.

HEAD HOME TO COMFORT FOODS

Sometimes a poor appetite can be remedied by those foods you adored during childhood: macaroni and cheese, mashed potatoes, green bean casserole, roast chicken, or a big slice of chocolate cake. A favorite dish or dessert can be just the cure you need to get yourself out of a digestive slump. Splurge on foods that make you feel better.

PREMENSTRUAL SYNDROME

Mood swings, along with a host of other symptoms such as water retention, breast swelling and tenderness, depression, irritability, fatigue, food cravings, and headaches, are known as premenstrual syndrome (PMS). They typically begin a few days to a week before menstruation and end when the menstrual period begins.

Researchers believe that about 40 percent of women of child-bearing age experience PMS in some form. Symptoms and severity vary from mild and manageable to severe and disruptive. Some women only have one symptom, while others have a whole constellation of symptoms. But PMS can be downright brutal for about 15 percent of women. They're the ones who experience many symptoms to a debilitating degree, causing serious problems on the job and in interpersonal relationships.

WHAT CAUSES PMS?

Doctors believe it is a result of hormonal changes, particularly in estrogen, that occur around the menstrual cycle. Some believe that PMS mood swings may be related to deficiencies in vitamin B6 and magnesium. One theory of PMS suggests that its symptoms are due to an ovarian hormone imbalance of either estrogen or progesterone.

Even though it's not fully understood, PMS is now recognized as a legitimate condition, not something that's all in women's heads. There are medications available that can mitigate or stop many of the harshest symptoms. Like so many other conditions, though, there are simple kitchen treatments that will work in relieving symptoms. So try them and see what happens. If you're a PMS sufferer, you know that anything that might help is worth a try.

KITCHEN CURES

AVOCADOS. These contain natural serotonin, which may supplement the mood-lifting brain chemical naturally produced by the body. Dates, plums, eggplants, papayas, plantains, and pineapple are also sources of serotonin.

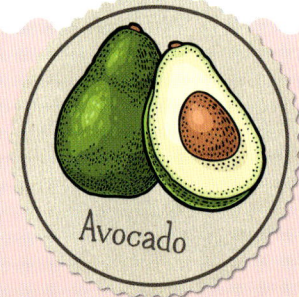
Avocado

BANANAS. Rich in potassium, they can relieve the bloating and swelling of water retention that comes with PMS. Other foods such as figs, black currants, potatoes, broccoli, onions, and tomatoes are potassium-rich, too.

BLACK PEPPER. Add a pinch to 1 tablespoon aloe vera gel, and take three times a day with meals to relieve symptoms such as backache and abdominal pain. Aloe vera gel taken with a pinch of cumin works well, too.

CHERRIES. An Ayurvedic remedy to relieve PMS symptoms, including bloating and mood swings, is to eat 10 fresh cherries on an empty stomach each day for one week before the start of the menstrual period.

CHICKEN. It's rich in vitamin B6, which may be depleted in women who suffer from PMS. Vitamin B6 may help relieve depression by raising levels of serotonin, a mood-enhancer, in the brain. Other B6-rich foods include fish, milk, brown rice, whole grains, soybeans, beans, walnuts, and green leafy vegetables.

CINNAMON. Good sleep habits are important in the treatment of PMS, and a brew of cinnamon tea is relaxing just before bed. Sweeten to taste with honey. Chamomile tea is a relaxing bedtime choice, too.

OATMEAL. It breaks down slowly and gradually releases sugar into the bloodstream. This slow, steady release combats the craving that comes with PMS. Rye bread, pasta, basmati rice, and fruit produce the same effect.

PASTA. This is enriched with magnesium, which is important for normal hormonal function. A lack of magnesium may be the cause of muscle cramps. Other magnesium-rich foods include green vegetables, breakfast cereals (skip those sugary ones), and potatoes.

SUNFLOWER SEEDS. They're rich in omega-6 fatty acid, which may be missing in women who suffer with PMS. Pumpkin and sesame seeds are also rich in it.

TURKEY. It supplies tryptophan, an amino acid that converts into serotonin, a mood-enhancer. Cottage cheese is another source of tryptophan.

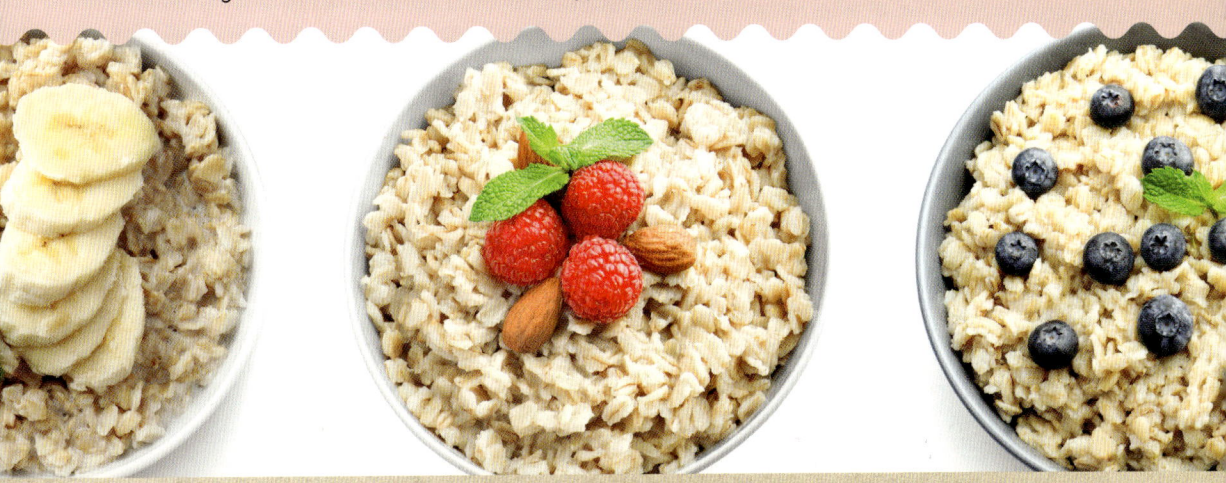

MORE DO'S & DON'TS

- **Forgo fats.** They may make PMS symptoms worse. Limit fat to less than 20 percent of your daily calories. Here's how to do the math:

  1. Divide your average daily calories by 5: If you eat 2,000 calories a day, that's 400.
  2. Divide that by 9. There are 9 calories per gram of fat: That comes to about 44 grams of fat allowed each day.

- **Crunch on carbs.** Fresh fruits, vegetables, and whole-grain cereals and breads can reduce the cravings that come with PMS. They also help elevate mood. Eat smaller meals, then snack on these carbohydrates every three hours: popcorn (skip the butter), pretzels, rice cakes. Consume about 100 calories per snack.

- **Cut the caffeine.** And that goes for coffee, cola, and chocolate. Caffeine contributes to breast pain and anxiety, two of the leading PMS complaints.

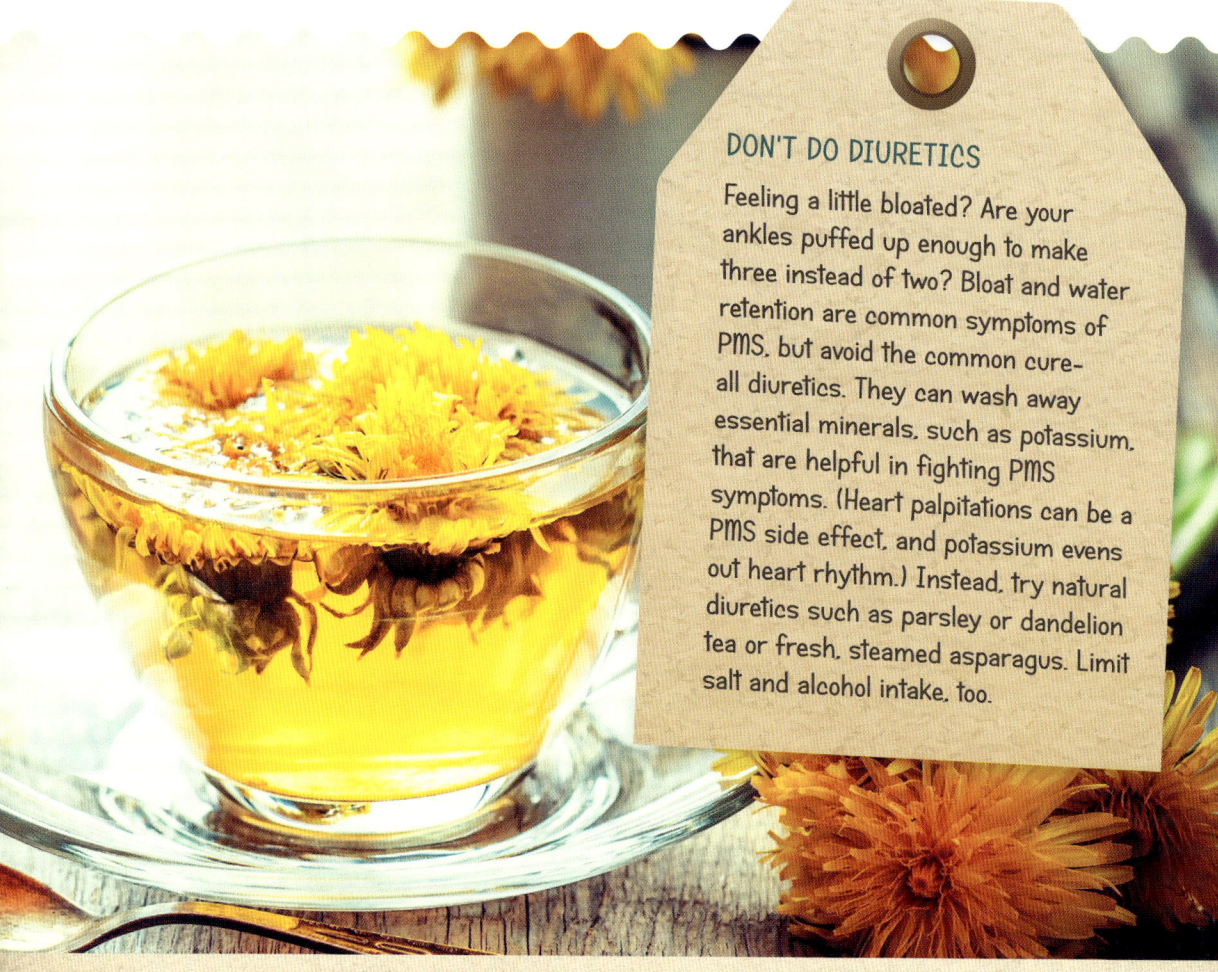

DON'T DO DIURETICS

Feeling a little bloated? Are your ankles puffed up enough to make three instead of two? Bloat and water retention are common symptoms of PMS, but avoid the common cure-all diuretics. They can wash away essential minerals, such as potassium, that are helpful in fighting PMS symptoms. (Heart palpitations can be a PMS side effect, and potassium evens out heart rhythm.) Instead, try natural diuretics such as parsley or dandelion tea or fresh, steamed asparagus. Limit salt and alcohol intake, too.

SEASONAL AFFECTIVE DISORDER

Ho hum. Another day, so much to do. But you can't seem to drag yourself out of bed. In fact, only thing you'd really like to do is snuggle in between the covers for a long winter's nap.

If that's a description of the way you feel every winter, you could be suffering from seasonal affective disorder, or SAD. It's a poorly understood condition that affects some people during the winter months, when there is less sunlight. In addition to a depressed mood, symptoms of SAD include cravings for carbohydrates, inability to concentrate, irritability, lethargy, weight gain, and a lack of interest in sex.

Doctors often treat SAD with antidepressants. For some, they work. For others, the side effects are overwhelming, often worse than the SAD itself. So if you've got SAD, look in the kitchen for some relief. Many of these raise your levels of serotonin, a substance that can help regulate mood levels.

KITCHEN CURES

APRICOTS. This fruit gradually raises serotonin levels and helps keep them there, as do apples, pears, grapes, plums, grapefruits, and oranges.

AVOCADOS. They are high in natural serotonin, which seems to suppress appetite. Also high in natural serotonin are dates, bananas, plums, eggplant, papayas, passion fruit, plantains, pineapples, and tomatoes.

BASMATI RICE. The sugar in this rice is slow to release into the bloodstream, which helps blood sugar levels stay constant instead of going through highs and lows. Drastic changes in blood sugar can lead to weight gain, which is a side effect of SAD. Other foods with a similar effect on blood sugar are rye bread and pasta.

BOUILLON. When the carbohydrate craving is just about to defeat you, drink some hot bouillon or broth. Hot liquids in the belly are filling, and consuming them before a meal is an old diet trick that reduces food consumption. Better the bouillon than the banana cream pie.

CEREALS. Cooked cereal, unsweetened muesli, and bran flakes are slow to release sugar into the bloodstream, which helps raise serotonin levels.

COTTAGE CHEESE. It's high in tryptophan, which is lacking in people with SAD. Other foods just as high in tryptophan are turkey, fish, and eggs.

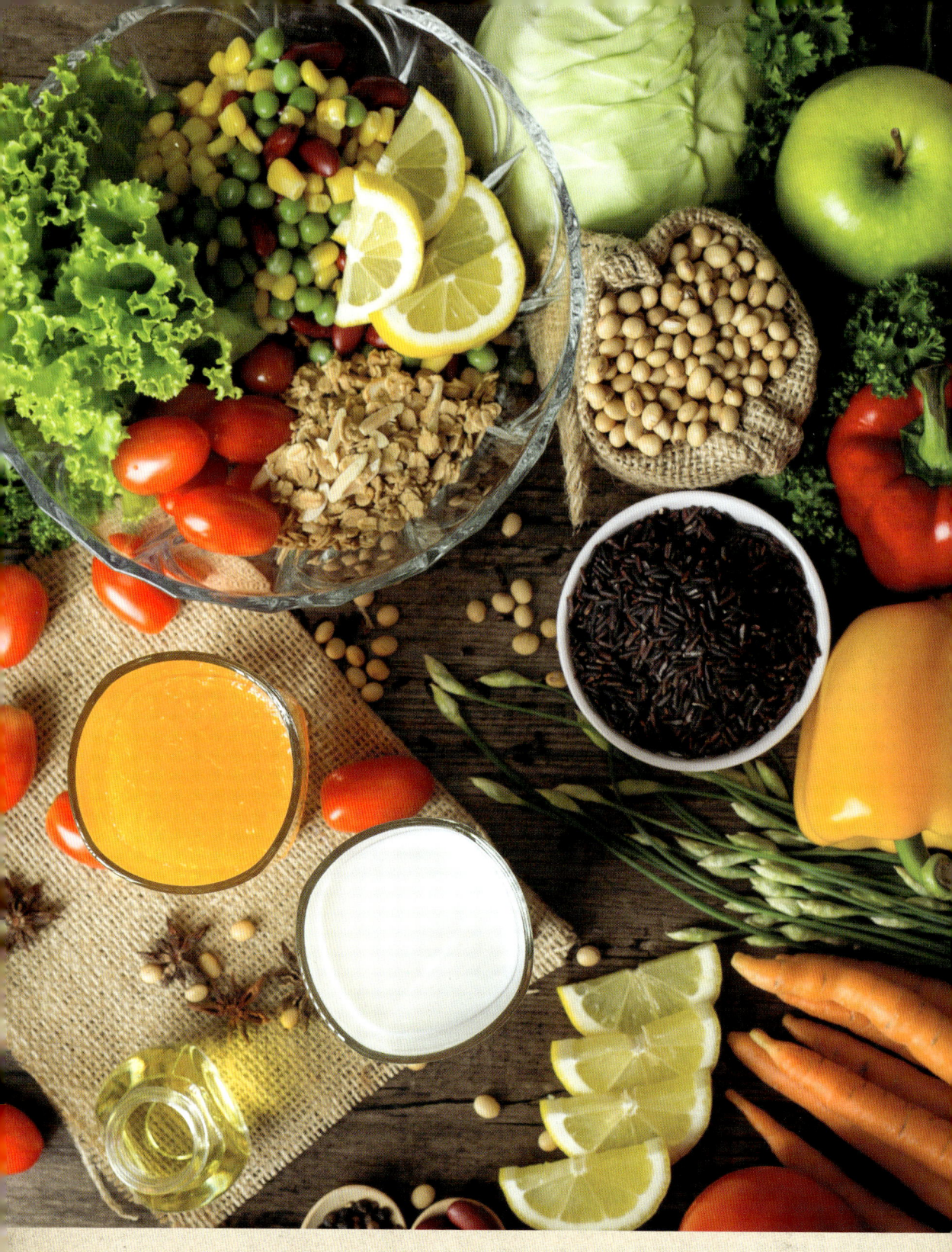

HERBAL TEAS. Any herbal tea is a better choice than teas with caffeine. Your reduced energy level may cause you to turn to caffeine for a boost, but it can also cause anxiety, muscle tension, and stomach problems, so opt for herbal. Chamomile, peppermint, and cinnamon are pleasant-tasting choices. Drink a cup instead of giving in to your carbohydrate cravings.

LEGUMES. These help maintain an even serotonin level throughout the day and night.

SHELLFISH. These are high in tyrosine, which forms chemicals that act on the brain cells to improve concentration and alertness, both of which become sluggish with SAD. Other foods high in tyrosine are fish, chicken, skinless turkey, cottage cheese, plain yogurt, skim milk, eggs, tofu, and very lean ham, pork, and lamb.

TURKEY. Protein foods such as turkey, low fat cottage cheese, chicken, and low fat dairy products can reduce the carbohydrate cravings of SAD as well as control the weight gain that occurs during SAD months.

BAD SAD FOODS

Because overeating and weight gain often go hand-in-hand with SAD, you need to take extra care to avoid the foods that trigger carbohydrate cravings. Here's a list of some of the worst offenders and what they do:

- **Sweets:** Sugar, honey, soft drinks, cookies, candy, cake. These quickly raise blood sugar levels and provide a quick serotonin boost that falls off rapidly. When this happens, the brain wants another quick fix and you crave more. This can turn into a never-ending cycle, since the body wants a serotonin high all the time.

- **Simple Carbohydrates:** Bread, bagel, potatoes. Starchy foods also cause a rapid rise in blood sugar, which gives the brain its fast serotonin high, then drops you like a rock.

- **Fats:** Butter, margarine, oil, and fatty foods. These can cause the weight gain that accompanies SAD. Weight gain may also contribute to the depression associated with SAD.

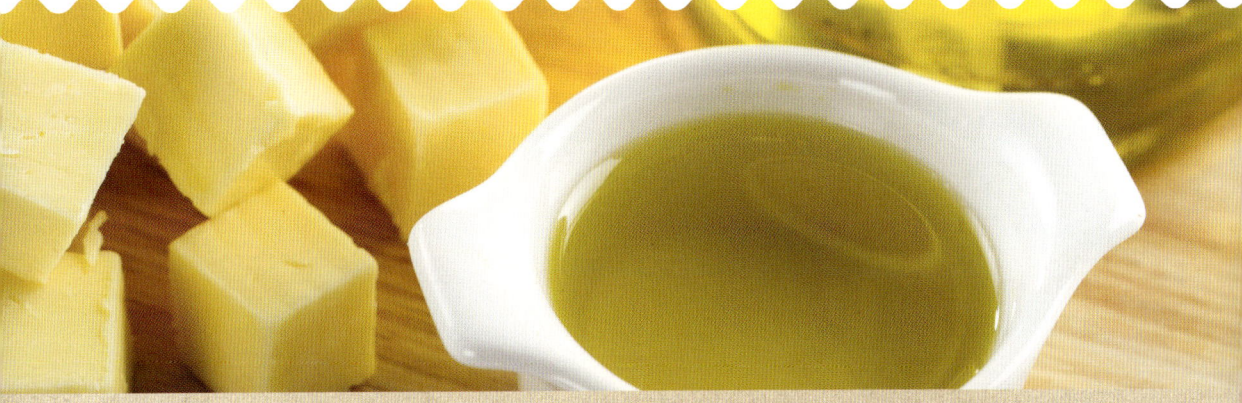

SORE THROAT

It's scratchy, tender, and swollen, and you dread the simple task of swallowing. But you must swallow, and when you do, you brace yourself for the unavoidable pain. If you've got a sore throat, you're in good company; everybody gets them, and 40 million people trek to the doctor's office for treatment of one every year.

The mechanics of a sore throat are pretty simple. It's an inflammation of the pharynx, which is the tube that extends from the back of the mouth to the esophagus. The following are the leading causes of sore throat:

- Viral infection (colds, flu, etc.). Often accompanied by fever, achy muscles, and runny nose, viral infections can't be cured but their symptoms can be treated. A sore throat from a viral source will generally disappear on its own within several days.
- Bacterial infection, especially from a streptococcal bacteria (strep throat). Symptoms are much like those of a viral infection but may be more severe and long lasting. Often a bacterial infection is accompanied by headache, stomachache, and swollen glands in the neck. A strep infection is generally treated with antibiotics because permanent heart or kidney damage can result. Culturing the bacteria is the only way a doctor can determine the cause of the sore throat.

While those are the primary reasons for a sore throat, there are others, including

- Smoking
- Acid reflux
- Allergies
- Dry air, especially at night when you may sleep with your mouth open
- Mouth breathing
- Throat abuse: singing, shouting, coughing
- Polyps or cancer
- Infected tonsils
- Food allergy

Whatever the cause, you want a cure when your throat's on fire. In some cases, medical attention is definitely required to cure the underlying infection. But there are soothing remedies to be found in the kitchen that can stand alone or work side-by-side with traditional medicine to stifle that soreness.

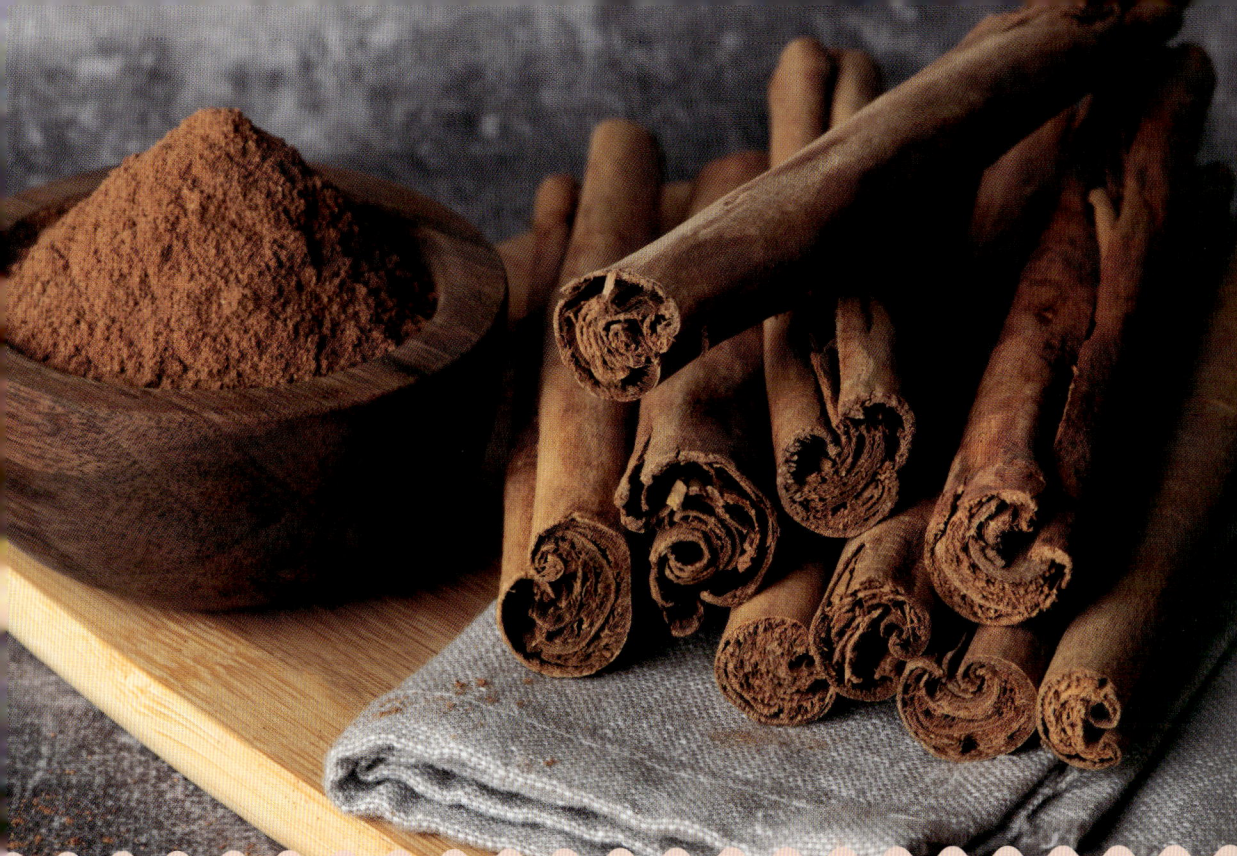

KITCHEN CURES

CINNAMON. Mix 2 parts cinnamon, 2 parts ginger, and 3 parts licorice powder. Steep 1 teaspoon of this mixture in 1 cup boiling water for ten minutes, then drink as a sore throat cure three times a day.

GARLIC. This Amish remedy can treat or prevent sore throats. Peel a fresh clove, slice it in half, and place 1 piece in each cheek. Suck on the garlic like a cough drop. Occasionally, crush your teeth against the garlic, not to bite it in half, but to release its allicin, a chemical that can kill the bacteria that causes strep.

HORSERADISH. Try this Russian sore throat cure. Combine 1 tablespoon pure horseradish or horseradish root with 1 teaspoon honey and 1 teaspoon ground cloves. Mix in a glass of warm water and drink slowly.

LEMON JUICE. Mix 1 tablespoon each of honey and lemon juice in 1 cup warm water. Sip this mixture.

LIME JUICE. Combine 1 spoonful with a spoonful of honey and take as often as needed for a sore throat.

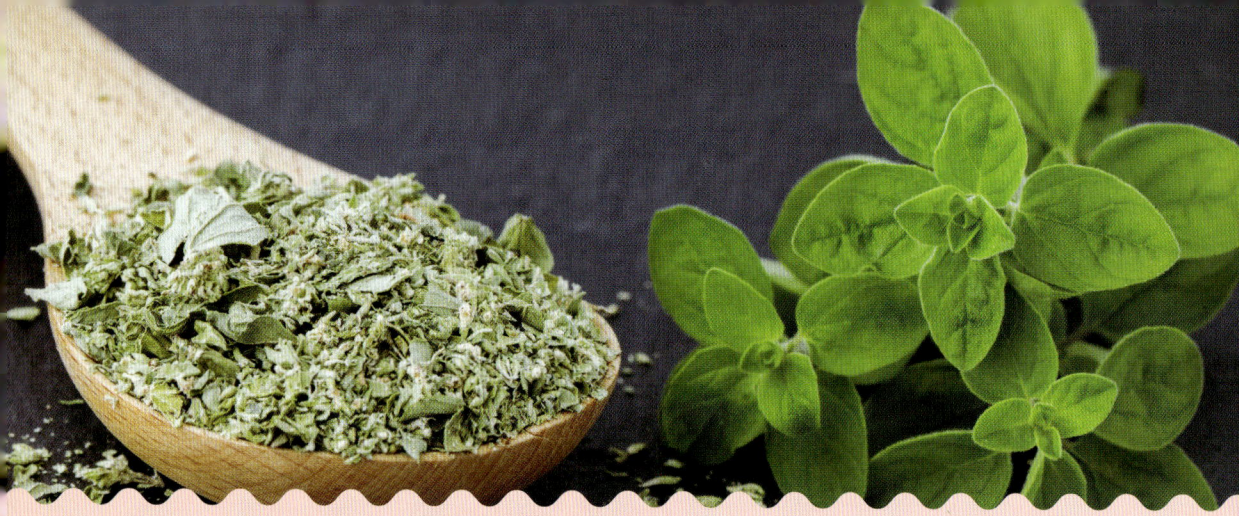

MARJORAM. Make a soothing tea with a spoonful of marjoram steeped in a cup of boiling water for ten minutes. Strain, then sweeten to taste with honey.

ONIONS. This tear-promoting veggie contains allicin, which can kill the bacteria that causes strep. Eat them raw or sautéed.

PEPPERMINT OIL. Add 2 drops each of peppermint and eucalyptus oils to 2 teaspoons olive oil and massage on the throat and upper chest for a nice, relaxing throat-soother.

SAGE. This curative herb is a great sore throat gargle. Mix 1 teaspoon in 1 cup boiling water. Steep for ten minutes, then strain. Add 1 teaspoon each cider vinegar and honey, then gargle four times a day.

TURMERIC. Try this gargle to calm a cranky throat. Mix together 1 cup hot water, ½ teaspoon turmeric, and ½ teaspoon salt. Gargle with the mixture twice a day. If you're not good with the gargle, mix ½ teaspoon turmeric in 1 cup hot milk and drink. Turmeric stains clothing, so be careful when mixing and gargling.

HERBAL CURES

CHAMOMILE. Make a tea by adding 1 teaspoon chamomile to 1 cup boiling water. Steep for ten minutes, strain, then gargle three to four times a day. Make a poultice by mixing 1 tablespoon chamomile flowers in 2 cups boiling water. Steep five minutes, then strain. Soak a clean towel in the warm solution, wring it out, and apply to throat. Remove when cold and reapply as often as necessary.

HOREHOUND. This is a great remedy for sore throats, but it's not a common herb found on most shelves. If you do happen to find it, make a tea with 1 tablespoon horehound leaves and 1 cup boiling water. Steep, strain, and gargle. Or, suck on some horehound hard candy.

STOMACH UPSET

When you eat something, the digestive process begins right away in your mouth. Your salivary glands produce digestive juices that lubricate your food and prepare fat for digestion. The food travels through your esophagus into your stomach, where digestive juices continue to break food down even further so it can travel on to the small intestine. The pancreas and liver secrete other digestive juices that flow into the small intestines. In the small intestine, vital nutrients including vitamins, minerals, water, salt, carbohydrates, and proteins are sucked out of the food and absorbed into your body. By the time your dinner makes its way to the large intestines, it's mostly bulk and water. The large intestines absorb the water and help you get rid of the, umm, excess.

But sometimes things in the digestive system go awry and cause indigestion, a catchall term that means you simply have trouble digesting your food. When you eat too much, or you eat the wrong foods, you may get one of a number of indigestion symptoms: nausea, vomiting, heartburn, bloating, or gas.

Those unpleasant feelings may send you running to the drugstore for relief, and if they do, you've got plenty of company. The American Gastroenterological Association says that digestive problems are one of the most common reasons Americans take over-the-counter medications. Indigestion can be a symptom of something more serious, such as gastritis, an ulcer, severe heartburn, irritable bowel syndrome, or diverticulitis. But if it's just the result of over-doing it at dinner, try some of these kitchen cures for relief.

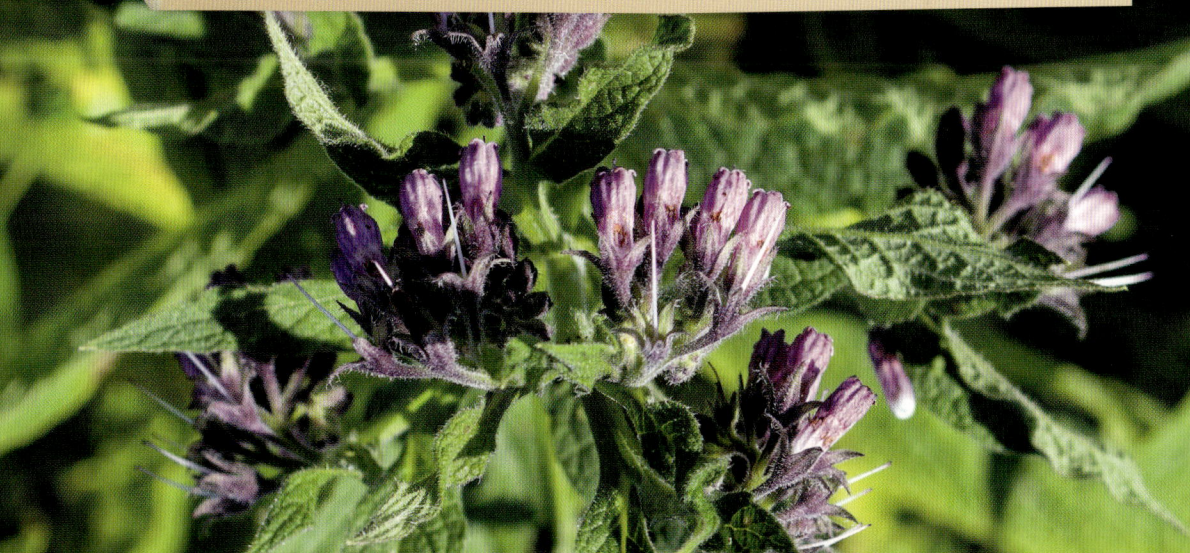

KITCHEN CURES

APPLE. Adding fiber to your diet will help alleviate stomachaches and keep your digestive system healthy. One study of fiber's effect on the tummy discovered that people who ate fiber-rich foods at the first sign of a tummyache cut their chances of getting a full-blown upset stomach in half. If you haven't been eating much fiber, be sure to start slowly. Jumping in with loads of fiber-rich foods after living on burgers and fries will give you a mean case of gas. Add fiber gradually over a few months and drink plenty of water to avoid overloading your system. To get started, grab an apple and nosh away, but remember to eat the peel—that's where you get most of your roughage.

BANANA. If you have a sensitive tummy, bland foods such as bananas seem to ease the pain. One study found that half the people who took banana powder capsules every day for two months eased their tummy pain. You can get similar results by eating a banana—or better yet a plantain banana—every day.

CARAWAY SEEDS. These seeds act very similarly to fennel seeds. They help with digestion and gas. You can either make a tea from the seed or you can do what people in Middle Eastern countries have done for centuries—simply chew on the seeds after dinner. Caraway seed tea: Place 1 teaspoon caraway seeds in a cup and add boiling water. Cover the cup and let stand for ten minutes. Strain well and drink up to 3 cups a day—be sure to drink on an empty stomach.

CINNAMON. This aromatic spice stimulates the digestive system, helping things move along the digestive tract smoothly. You can make a cinnamon tea by stirring ¼ to ½ teaspoon cinnamon powder into 1 cup hot water. Let the tea stand for up to five minutes and drink.

CRACKERS. You haven't eaten anything all day, and you can't understand why your stomach is churning and burning. The answer is probably overactive stomach acids. And your best bet is to eat something but to stick with something bland, such as nibbling on crackers.

FENNEL SEEDS. This remedy is one of the most prescribed for gas and stomach cramps by medical herbalists. Try a fennel tea for your stomach: Place 1 teaspoon fennel seeds in a cup and add boiling water. Cover the cup and let stand for ten minutes. Strain well and drink up to 3 cups a day—be sure to drink on an empty stomach.

GINGER. Ginger is a long-time helper for stomach ailments of all types—particularly nausea and gas. Ginger helps food flow smoothly through the digestive tract, allowing the body to better absorb nutrients. Drink a cup of ginger tea to get your stomach back on track. To make your own ginger tea: Add ½ teaspoon ground ginger to a cup of hot water, let stand for up to three minutes, strain, and drink away.

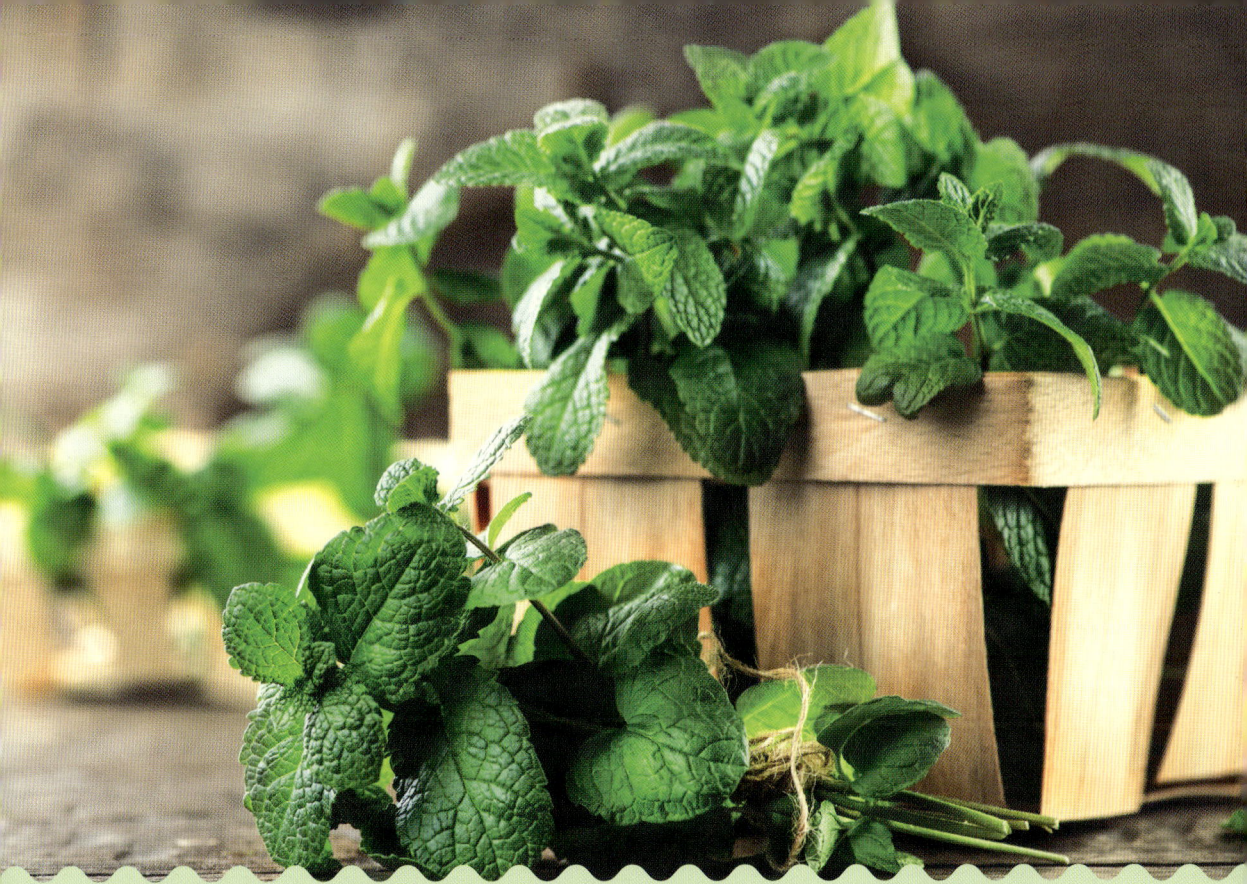

MINT. A folk remedy for indigestion, mint (in the form of peppermint or spearmint) can soothe a troubled tummy. Mint helps food move through the intestines properly and eases stomach cramps. Sip a cup of mint tea to let the herb work its magic: Put 1 teaspoon dried mint in a cup and add boiling water. Cover the cup and let it stand for ten minutes. Strain and drink up to 3 cups of the warm tea a day. Be sure to drink it on an empty stomach.

RICE. If an overflow of stomach acid bothers you, try eating ½ cup cooked rice with your dinner. It's a complex carbohydrate that keeps the stomach busy churning, diverting excess acid. Plus it's a bland food that tends to be easy on the stomach.

SODA POP. Sipping on a can of decaffeinated soda can help settle your stomach. This trick is especially useful if you've eaten too much. The carbonation in the soda causes you to burp, which is the quickest way to get relief from an overfull belly.

THYME. Thyme stimulates the digestive tract, helps with stomach cramping, and relieves gas pressure. Try some thyme in a bottle (or cup) for your tummy trouble: Place 1 teaspoon dried thyme leaves in a cup. Fill the cup with boiling water and let stand, covered, for ten minutes. Strain and drink on an empty stomach up to three times a day.

MORE DO'S AND DON'TS

- **Think twice about milk.** Though many people think milk can soothe an aching tummy, it actually may do more harm than good. People who are lactose intolerant have trouble digesting milk and end up with bloating, gas, and cramping.

- **Cut the coffee.** Coffee causes stomach irritation in some people.

- **Ax the alcohol.** Alcohol is also a stomach irritant. If you have a sensitive tummy, skip the after-dinner drink.

- **Pass on pepper.** Red or black pepper may add a kick to food, but it can also kick you in the tummy. Avoid it if it bothers your stomach.

- **Choose produce carefully.** Some vegetables and fruits are notorious for their ability to produce tummy trouble. Watch out for broccoli, cabbage, Brussels sprouts, and melons.

- **Wash your beans.** Beans are the "musical fruit," but you can take the music out of them. Let them soak overnight in water, then drain the water and replace it with fresh water before cooking. Rinse canned beans, too. This simple technique will help avert gassy problems.

- **Eat up.** Don't skip meals. It allows acid to build up in your stomach and can leave you with an aching tummy.

TROUBLESOME FOODS

German researchers wanted to know what foods caused the most trouble for people. So they asked people what foods tended to create an aching tummy. The top three offenders for normal, healthy eaters were mayonnaise, cabbage, and fried and salted foods.

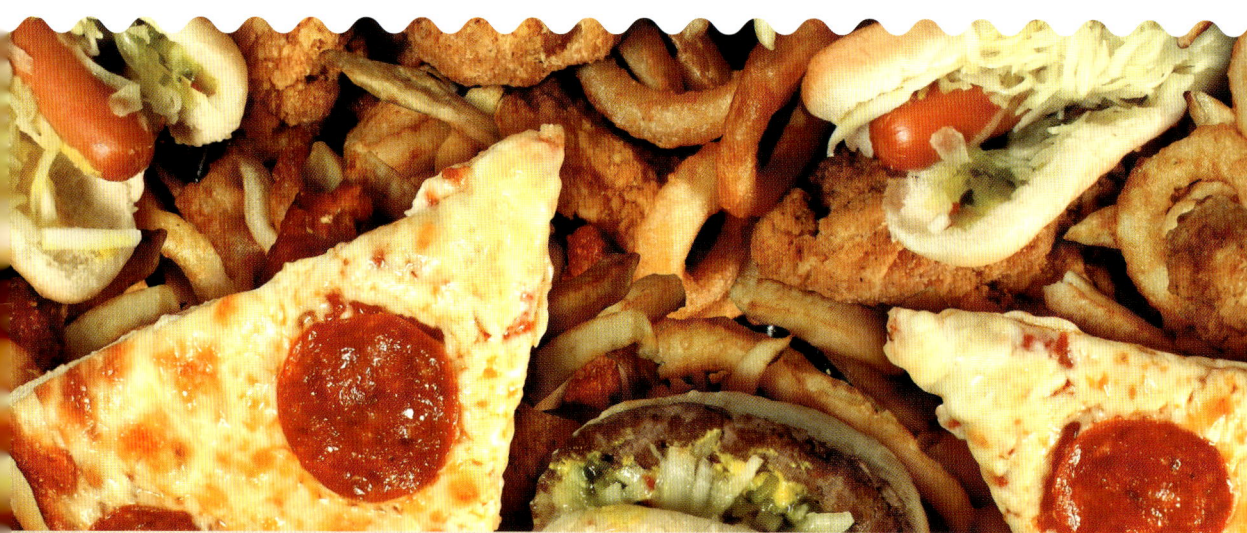

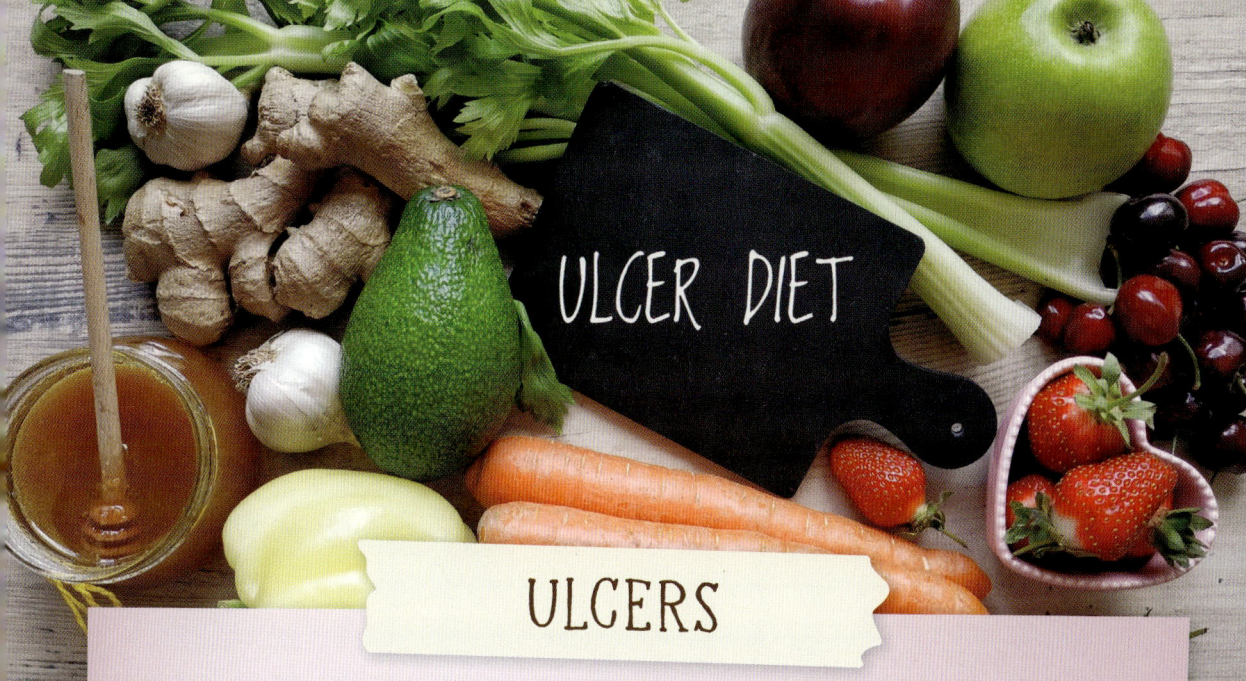

ULCERS

It's only in the last few decades that scientific evidence conclusively proved that ulcers are most often caused by a bacterial infection, not by the Type-A, pressure-cooker personality that was the subject of countless jokes. Misconceptions and myths die hard, though, so there are some people who haven't gotten the word yet and still believe that the demanding boss or the overachiever are more likely to work themselves into an ulcer. While these personality characteristics may aggravate an existing ulcer (not to mention the people they associate with), they don't cause one.

THERE'S A HOLE IN THE BUCKET

An ulcer is a sore or hole in the protective mucosal lining of the gastrointestinal tract. Ulcers appear in the area of the stomach or the duodenum, the upper part of the small intestine, where caustic digestive juices, pepsin, and hydrochloric acid are present. Today we know that the majority of ulcers are the result of an infection with a bacteria called *Helicobacter pylori (H. pylori)*. This bacteria makes the stomach and small intestine more susceptible to the erosive effects of the digestive juices. The bacteria may also cause the stomach to produce more acid.

There are some lifestyle factors that can contribute to the development of an ulcer. These include alcohol consumption, eating and drinking foods that contain caffeine, significant physical (not emotional) stress such as severe burns and major surgery, and excessive use of certain over-the-counter pain medications such as aspirin or ibuprofen. Studies have shown that smoking also tends to increase the chances of developing an ulcer, slows the healing of existing ulcers, and makes a recurrence more likely. Family history of ulcers also appears to play a role in susceptibility.

WHO GETS ULCERS?

If Type-A folks don't automatically get ulcers, then who does? The cause lies less in personality and more in stomach makeup. Researchers believe some people just produce more stomach acid than others. If stomach acid production isn't the problem, then a weak stomach may be. The stomach lining in certain individuals may be less able to withstand the onslaught of gastric acids. Lifestyle factors mentioned above can also weaken the stomach's lining.

SIGNS AND SYMPTOMS

You're probably familiar with the most typical symptom of a brewing ulcer: a burning or gnawing pain between the breastbone and navel. This pain is more common between meals (it improves with eating but returns a few hours later) and in the middle of the night or toward dawn.

Less typical symptoms include nausea or vomiting, weight loss and loss of appetite, and frequent burping or bloating.

If you have an ulcer or suspect you may have one, you should be under the care of a physician. But between visits to the doctor, there are ways to care for your digestive tract.

FOOD SURPRISES

Milk was an early treatment for ulcer flare-ups, but it is no longer considered a good drink if you have ulcers. Foods high in calcium, such as milk, stimulate stomach acid. Limit your milk intake according to your doctor's advice.

Highly spiced and fried foods, on the other hand, once were thought to be prime culprits in starting ulcers. But research has shown that they have little or no bearing either on the development or the course of an ulcer. This is not to say that such food won't cause irritation. Watch what you pull from the refrigerator and note your gut reaction to each. If you experience discomfort, ban the food from the fridge. If nothing happens after popping that pizza slice into your pouch—rejoice and enjoy!

KITCHEN CURES

BANANAS. These fruits contain an antibacterial substance that may inhibit the growth of ulcer-causing *H. pylori*. And studies show that animals fed bananas have a thicker stomach wall and greater mucus production in the stomach, which helps build a better barrier between digestive acids and the lining of the stomach. Eating plantains is also helpful.

CABBAGE. Researchers have found that ulcer patients who drink 1 quart of raw cabbage juice a day can often heal their ulcers in five days. If chugging a quart of cabbage juice turns your stomach inside out, researchers also found that those who eat plain cabbage have quicker healing times as well. Time for some coleslaw!

CAYENNE PEPPER. Used moderately, a little cayenne pepper can go a long way in helping ulcers. The pepper stimulates blood flow to bring nutrients to the stomach. To make a cup of peppered tea, mix ¼ teaspoon cayenne pepper in 1 cup hot water. Drink a cup a day. A dash of cayenne pepper can also be added to soups, meats, and other savory dishes.

GARLIC. Garlic's antibacterial properties include fighting *H. pylori*. Take two small crushed cloves a day.

LICORICE. Several modern studies have demonstrated the ulcer-healing abilities of licorice. Licorice does its part not by reducing stomach acid but rather by reducing the ability of stomach acid to damage stomach lining. Properties in licorice encourage digestive mucosal tissues to protect themselves from acid. Licorice can be used in encapsulated form, but for a quick cup of licorice tea, cut 1 ounce licorice root into slices and cover with 1 quart boiling water. Steep, cool, and strain. (If licorice root is unavailable, cut 1 ounce licorice sticks into slices.) You can also try licorice candy if it's made with real licorice (the label will say "licorice mass") and not just flavored with anise. Don't eat more than 1 ounce per day.

PLUMS. Red- and purple-colored foods inhibit the growth of *H. pylori*. Like plums, berries too can help you fight the good fight.

URINARY TRACT INFECTION

You stand in front of the bathroom door for the twentieth time in the last hour. You've got to go, but every time you do, you end up with only a painful trickle. You recognize the burning sensation that makes every trip to the toilet an ordeal. You've got a urinary tract infection.

Urinary tract infections (UTIs) are the second most common reason people visit their doctors each year. Men get UTIs, but they are much more common in women. If you've ever had a UTI, you'll probably never forget the symptoms. It usually starts with a sudden and frequent need to visit the potty. When you get there, you can squeeze out only a little bit of urine, and that's usually accompanied by a burning sensation in your bladder and/or urethra. In more extreme cases you may end up with fever, chills, back pain, and even blood in your urine.

UTIs that last longer than two days require medical intervention. Untreated UTIs can infect the kidneys and turn into a much more serious problem. To help prevent a UTI from developing or nip one in the bud, try some of the remedies available in your own kitchen.

KITCHEN CURES

BLUEBERRIES. Blueberries and cranberries are from the same plant family and seem to have the same bacteria-inhibiting properties. In one study, blueberry juice was found to prevent UTIs. Since you're not likely to find a gallon of blueberry juice at your local store, try sprinkling a handful of these flavorful, good-for-you berries over your morning cereal.

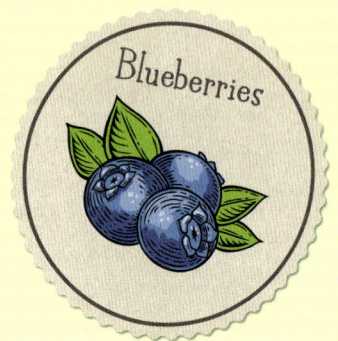

CRANBERRY JUICE. Many studies have found that drinking cranberry juice may help you avoid urinary tract infections. It appears that cranberry juice prevents infection-causing bacteria from bedding down in your bladder, and it also has a very mild antibiotic affect. Drinking as little as 4 ounces of cranberry juice a day can help keep your bladder infection-free. But if you tend to get UTIs or are dealing with one right now, try to drink at least 2 to 4 glasses of cranberry juice a day. If pure cranberry juice is just too bitter for your taste buds, you can substitute cranberry juice cocktail. It seems to have the same effect as the pure stuff. Take note: If you have a UTI, cranberry juice is not a replacement for doctor-prescribed antibiotics in treating your infection.

PINEAPPLE. Bromelain is an enzyme found in pineapples. In one study, people with a UTI who were given bromelain along with their usual round of antibiotics got rid of their infection. Only half the people who were given a placebo plus an antibiotic showed no signs of lingering infection. Eating a cup of pineapple tastes good and may just help rid you of your infection.

VITAMIN C. Some doctors are prescribing at least 5,000 mg or more of vitamin C a day for patients who develop recurrent urinary tract infections. Vitamin C keeps the bladder healthy by acidifying the urine, essentially putting up a no-trespassing sign for potentially harmful bacteria.

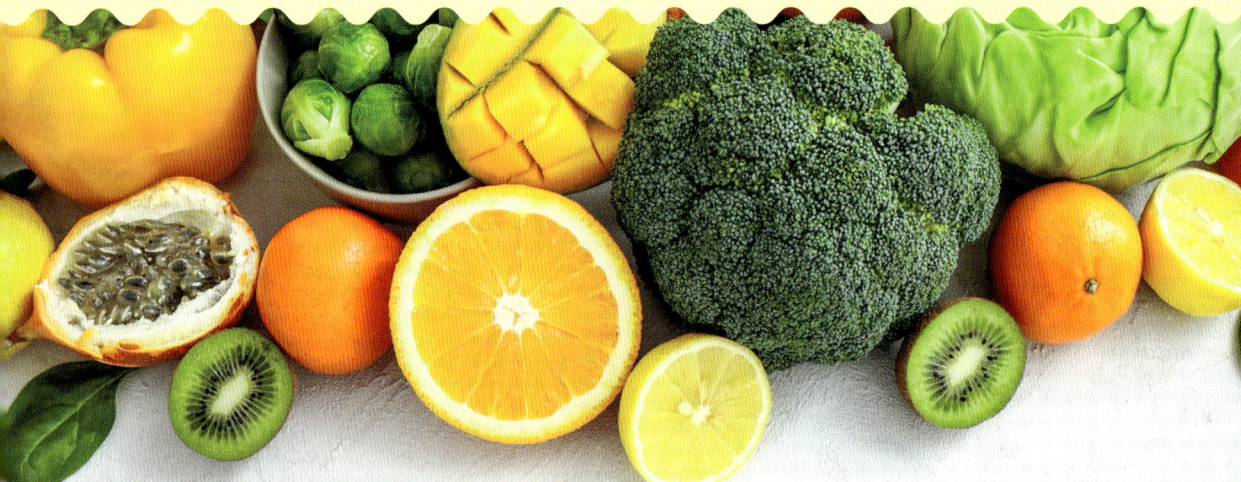